Multiple Comparisons Using R

Multiple Comparisons Using R

Frank Bretz
Torsten Hothorn
Peter Westfall

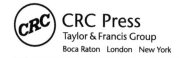

CRC Press
Taylor & Francis Group
Boca Raton London New York

CRC Press is an imprint of the
Taylor & Francis Group an **informa** business

A CHAPMAN & HALL BOOK

Chapman & Hall/CRC
Taylor & Francis Group
6000 Broken Sound Parkway NW, Suite 300
Boca Raton, FL 33487-2742

© 2011 by Taylor and Francis Group, LLC
Chapman & Hall/CRC is an imprint of Taylor & Francis Group, an Informa business

No claim to original U.S. Government works

International Standard Book Number: 978-1-58488-574-0 (Hardback)

Library of Congress Cataloging-in-Publication Data

Bretz, Frank.
    Multiple comparisons using R / Frank Bretz, Torsten Hothorn, Peter Westfall.
       p. cm.
    Includes bibliographical references and index.
    ISBN 978-1-58488-574-0 (hardcover : alk. paper)
    1. Multiple comparisons (Statistics) 2. R (Computer program language) I. Hothorn, Torsten. II. Westfall, Peter H., 1957- III. Title.

QA278.4.B74 2011
519.5--dc22   2010023538

Visit the Taylor & Francis Web site at
http://www.taylorandfrancis.com

and the CRC Press Web site at
http://www.crcpress.com

To Jiamei and my parents
— F.B.

To Carolin, Elke and Ludwig
— T.H.

To Marilyn and Amy
— P.W.

Contents

List of Figures ix

List of Tables xi

Preface xiii

1 Introduction 1

2 General Concepts 11
  2.1 Error rates and general concepts 11
    2.1.1 Error rates 11
    2.1.2 General concepts 17
  2.2 Construction methods 20
    2.2.1 Union intersection test 20
    2.2.2 Intersection union test 22
    2.2.3 Closure principle 23
    2.2.4 Partitioning principle 29
  2.3 Methods based on Bonferroni's inequality 31
    2.3.1 Bonferroni test 31
    2.3.2 Holm procedure 32
    2.3.3 Further topics 34
  2.4 Methods based on Simes' inequality 35

3 Multiple Comparisons in Parametric Models 41
  3.1 General linear models 41
    3.1.1 Multiple comparisons in linear models 41
    3.1.2 The linear regression example revisited using R 45
  3.2 Extensions to general parametric models 48
    3.2.1 Asymptotic results 48
    3.2.2 Multiple comparisons in general parametric models 50
    3.2.3 Applications 52
  3.3 The **multcomp** package 53
    3.3.1 The `glht` function 53
    3.3.2 The `summary` method 59
    3.3.3 The `confint` method 64

4 Applications   **69**

4.1 Multiple comparisons with a control   70

    4.1.1 Dunnett test   71

    4.1.2 Step-down Dunnett test procedure   77

4.2 All pairwise comparisons   82

    4.2.1 Tukey test   82

    4.2.2 Closed Tukey test procedure   93

4.3 Dose response analyses   99

    4.3.1 A dose response study on litter weight in mice   100

    4.3.2 Trend tests   103

4.4 Variable selection in regression models   108

4.5 Simultaneous confidence bands   111

4.6 Multiple comparisons under heteroscedasticity   114

4.7 Multiple comparisons in logistic regression models   118

4.8 Multiple comparisons in survival models   124

4.9 Multiple comparisons in mixed-effects models   125

5 Further Topics   **127**

5.1 Resampling-based multiple comparison procedures   127

    5.1.1 Permutation methods   127

    5.1.2 Using R for permutation multiple testing   137

    5.1.3 Bootstrap testing – Brief overview   140

5.2 Group sequential and adaptive designs   140

    5.2.1 Group sequential designs   141

    5.2.2 Adaptive designs   150

5.3 Combining multiple comparisons with modeling   156

    5.3.1 MCP-Mod: Dose response analyses under model uncertainty   157

    5.3.2 A dose response example   162

Bibliography   **167**

Index   **183**

List of Figures

1.1   Probability of committing at least one Type I error   2
1.2   Scatter plot of the thuesen data   4
1.3   Impact of multiplicity on selection bias   8

2.1   Visualization of two null hypotheses in the parameter space   24
2.2   Venn-type diagram for two null hypotheses   25
2.3   Schematic diagram of the closure principle for two null
      hypotheses   25
2.4   Schematic diagram of the closure principle for three null
      hypotheses   27
2.5   Partitioning principle for two null hypotheses   30
2.6   Schematic diagram of the closure principle for three null
      hypotheses under the restricted combination condition   33
2.7   Rejection regions for the Bonferroni and Simes tests   36
2.8   Power comparison for the Bonferroni and Simes tests   37

3.1   Boxplots of the warpbreaks data   54
3.2   Two-sided simultaneous confidence intervals for the Tukey
      test in the warpbreaks example   65
3.3   Compact letter display for all pairwise comparisons in the
      warpbreaks example   67

4.1   Boxplots of the recovery data   70
4.2   One-sided simultaneous confidence intervals for the Dunnett
      test in the recovery example   76
4.3   Closed Dunnett test in the recovery example   81
4.4   Two-sided simultaneous confidence intervals for the Tukey
      test in the immer example   87
4.5   Compact letter display for all pairwise comparisons in the
      immer example   89
4.6   Alternative compact letter display for all pairwise comparisons
      in the immer example   90
4.7   Mean-mean multiple comparison and tiebreaker plot for all
      pairwise comparisons in the immer example   92
4.8   Mean-mean multiple comparison plot for selected orthogonal
      contrasts in the immer example   94

4.9   Schematic diagram of the closure principle for all pairwise
        comparisons of four means   96
4.10   Summary plot of the Thalidomide dose response study   102
4.11   Plot of contrast coefficients for the Williams and modified
        Williams tests   105
4.12   Simultaneous confidence band for the difference of two linear
        regression models   114
4.13   Boxplots of alpha synuclein mRNA expression levels   115
4.14   Comparison of simultaneous confidence intervals based on
        different estimates of the covariance matrix   119
4.15   Association between smoking behavior and disease status
        stratified by gender   121
4.16   Simultaneous confidence intervals for the probability of
        suffering from Alzheimer's disease   123
4.17   Layout of the `trees513` field experiment   125
4.18   Probability of roe deer browsing damage   126

5.1   Schematic diagram of the closed hypotheses set for the
        adverse event data   130
5.2   Histograms of hypergeometric distributions   132
5.3   Wang-Tsiatis boundary examples   143
5.4   Hwang-Shih-DeCani spending function examples   144
5.5   Stopping boundaries for group sequential design example   147
5.6   Power plots for group sequential design example   149
5.7   Average sample sizes for group sequential design example   150
5.8   Schematic diagram of the closure principle for testing adap-
        tively two null hypotheses   153
5.9   Disjunctive power for different adaptive design options   156
5.10   Schematic overview of the MCP-Mod procedure   158
5.11   Model shapes for the selected candidate model set   164
5.12   Fitted model for the `biom` data   166

List of Tables

2.1   Type I and Type II errors in multiple hypotheses testing   12

2.2   Comparison of the Holm and Hochberg procedures   39

3.1   Multiple comparison procedures available in **multcomp**   62

4.1   Comparison of several multiple comparison procedures for the `recovery` data   82

4.2   Comparison of several multiple comparison procedures for the `immer` data   100

4.3   Summary data of the Thalidomide dose response example   101

4.4   Summary of the `alzheimer` data   120

5.1   Mock-up adverse event data   128

5.2   Adverse event contingency tables   131

5.3   Upper-tailed p-values for Fisher's exact test   133

5.4   Mock-up dataset with four treatment groups   136

5.5   Summary results of a study with two treatments and four outcome variables   139

5.6   Dose response models implemented in the **DoseFinding** package   160

Preface

Many scientific experiments subject to rigorous statistical analyses involve the simultaneous evaluation of more than one question. Multiplicity therefore becomes an inherent problem with various unintended consequences. The most widely recognized result is that the findings of an experiment can be misleading: Seemingly significant effects occur more often than expected by chance alone and not compensating for multiplicity can have important real world consequences. For instance, when the multiple comparisons involve drug efficacy, they may result in approval of a drug as an improvement over existing drugs, when there is in fact no beneficial effect. On the other hand, when drug safety is involved, it could happen by chance that the new drug appears to be worse for some side effect, when it is actually not worse at all. By contrast, multiple comparison procedures adjust statistical inferences from an experiment for multiplicity. Multiple comparison procedures thus enable better decision making and prevent the experimenter from declaring an effect when there is none.

Other books on multiple comparison procedures

There are different ways to approach the subject of multiple comparison procedures. Hochberg and Tamhane (1987) provided an extensive mathematical treatise on this topic. Westfall and Young (1993) focused on resampling-based multiple test approaches that incorporate stochastic dependencies in the data. Another approach is to introduce multiple comparison procedures by comparison type (multiple comparisons with a control, multiple comparisons with the best, etc.), as done in Hsu (1996). Westfall, Tobias, Rom, Wolfinger, and Hochberg (1999) chose an example-based approach, starting with simple problems and progressing to more challenging applications while introducing new methodology as needed. Dudoit and van der Laan (2008) described multiple comparison procedures relevant to genomics. Finally, Dmitrienko, Tamhane, and Bretz (2009) reviewed multiple comparison procedures used in pharmaceutical statistics by focusing on different drug development applications.

How is this book different?

The emphasis of this book is similar to the previous books in the development of the theory, but differs in the way that applications of multiple comparison procedures are presented. Too often, potential users of these methods are overwhelmed by the bewildering number of possible approaches. We adopt a unifying theme based on maximum statistics that, for example, shows Dunnett's and Tukey's methods to be essentially no different. This theme is emphasized throughout the book, as we describe the common underlying theory of multiple comparison procedures by use of several examples. In addition, we give a detailed description of available software implementations in R, a language and environment for statistical computing and graphics (Ihaka and Gentleman 1996). This book thus provides a self-contained introduction to multiple comparison procedures, with discussion and analysis of many examples using available software. In this book we focus on "classical" applications of multiple comparison procedures, where the number of comparisons is moderate and/or where strong evidence is needed.

How to read this book

In Chapter 1 we discuss the *"difficult and ubiquitous problems of multiplicity"* (Berry 2007). We give several characterizations and provide examples to motivate the discussion in the subsequent chapters. In Chapter 2 we give a general introduction to multiple hypotheses testing. We describe different error rates and introduce standard terminology. We also cover basic multiple comparison procedures, including the Bonferroni method and the Simes test. Chapter 3 provides the theoretical framework for the applications in Chapter 4. We briefly review standard linear model theory and show how to perform multiple comparisons in this framework. The resulting methods require the common analysis-of-variance assumptions and thus extend the basic approaches of Bonferroni and Simes. We then extend this framework and consider multiple comparison procedures in parametric models relying only on standard asymptotic normality assumptions. We further give a detailed introduction to the **multcomp** package in R, which provides a convenient interface to perform multiple comparisons in this general context. Applications to illustrate the results from this chapter are given in Chapter 4. Examples include the Dunnett test, Tukey's all-pairwise comparisons, and general multiple contrast tests, both for one-way layouts as well as for more complicated models with factorial treatment structures and/or covariates. We also give examples using mixed-effects models and applications to survival data. Finally, we review in Chapter 5 a selection of further multiple comparison procedures, which do not quite fit into the framework of Chapters 3 and 4. This includes the comparison of means with two-sample multivariate data using resampling-based procedures, methods for group sequential or adaptive designs, and the combination of multiple comparison procedures with modeling techniques.

Those who are facing multiple comparison problems for the first time might want to glance through Chapter 2, skip the detailed theoretical framework of Chapter 3 and proceed directly to the applications in Chapter 4. The quick reader may start with Chapter 4, which can be read mostly on its own; necessary theoretical results are linked backwards to Chapters 2 and 3. Similarly, the selected multiple comparison procedures in Chapter 5 can be read without necessarily having read the previous chapters.

Who should read this book

This book is for statistics teachers and students, undergraduate or graduate, who are learning about multiple comparison procedures, whether in a stand-alone course on multiple testing, a course in analysis-of-variance, a course in multivariate analysis, or a course in nonparameterics. Additionally, the book is helpful for scientists who need to use multiple comparison procedures, including biometricians, clinicians, medical doctors, molecular biologists, agricultural analysts, etc. It is oriented towards users (i) who have only limited knowledge of multiple comparison procedures but need to apply those techniques in R, and (ii) who are already familiar with multiple comparison procedures but lack the related implementations in R. We assume that the reader has a basic knowledge of R and can perform elementary data handling steps. Otherwise, we recommend standard textbooks on R for a quick introduction; see Dalgaard (2002) and Everitt and Hothorn (2009) among others.

Conventions used in this book

We use bold-face capital letters (e.g., $\mathbf{C}, \mathbf{R}, \mathbf{X}, \ldots$) to denote matrices and bold-face small letters (e.g., $\mathbf{c}, \mathbf{x}, \mathbf{y}, \ldots$) to indicate vectors. If the distinction between column and row vectors matters, we introduce vectors as column vectors. A transpose of a vector or matrix is indicated by the superscript $^\top$; for example, $\mathbf{c}^\top$ denotes the transpose of the (column) vector $\mathbf{c}$. To simplify the notation, we do not distinguish between random variables and their observed values, unless noted explicitly.

We use many code examples in R throughout this book. Samples of code that could be entered interactively at the R command line are formatted as follows:

```
R> library("multcomp")
```

Here, R> denotes the prompt sign from the R command line and the user enters everything else. In some instances the expressions to be entered will be longer than a single line and it will appear as follows:

```
R> summary(glht(recovery.aov, linfct = mcp(blanket = contr),
+               alternative = "less"))
```

The symbol + indicates additional lines which are appropriately indented. Finally, output produced by function calls is shown below the associated code

```
R> rnorm(10)
 [1]  0.0310  1.3378  0.4158  0.0413 -1.4383  1.0761 -1.2687
 [8]  0.8262 -0.8603 -0.7134
```

Computational details and reproducibility

In this book, we use several R packages to access different example datasets (such as **ISwR**, **MASS**, etc.), standard functions for the general parametric analyses (such as aov, lm, nlme, etc.) and the **multcomp** package to perform the multiple comparsion procedures. All of the packages used in this book are available at the Comprehensive R Archive Network (CRAN), which can be accessed from http://CRAN.R-project.org.

The source code for the analyses presented in this book is available from the **multcomp** package. A demo containing the R code to reproduce the individual results is available for each chapter by invoking

```
R> library("multcomp")
R> demo("Ch_Intro")
R> demo("Ch_Theory")
R> demo("Ch_GLM")
R> demo("Ch_Appl")
R> demo("Ch_Misc")
```

The results presented in this book and obtained with the **multcomp** package in general have been validated to the extent possible against the SAS macros described in Westfall et al. (1999). The **multcomp** package also includes SAS code for most of the examples presented in Chapters 1, 3 and 4. It can be accessed in R via

```
R> file.show(system.file("MCMT", "multcomp.sas",
+                        package = "multcomp"))
```

Readers should not expect to get exactly the same results as stated in this book. For example, differences in random number generating seeds or truncating the number of significant digits in the results may result in slight differences to the output shown here.

Acknowledgments

This book started as a presentation at the 2004 UseR! conference in Vienna, Austria. Many individuals have influenced the writing of this book since then. Our joint work over many years with Werner Brannath, Edgar Brunner, Alan Genz, Ekkehard Glimm, Gerhard Hommel, Ludwig Hothorn, Jason Hsu, Franz König, Willi Maurer, José Pinheiro, Martin Posch, Stephen Senn, Klaus Strassburger, Ajit Tamhane, Randy Tobias, and James Troendle had a direct impact on this book and we are grateful for the many fruitful discussions. We are indebted to Sylvia Davis and Kevin Henning for their close reading and criticism of an earlier version of this book. Their comments and suggestions have greatly improved the presentation of the material. Björn Bornkamp, Richard Heiberger, Wei Liu, Hans-Peter Piepho, and Gernot Wassmer read sections of the manuscript and provided much needed help during the progress of this book. We are especially indebted to Richard Heiberger who, over many years, provided valuable feedback on new functionality in **multcomp** and donated code to this project. Achim Zeileis gave suggestions on the new user interface and was, is, and hopefully will continue being someone to discuss computational and other problems with. André Schützenmeister developed the code for producing compact letter displays in **multcomp**. We also thank the book's acquisitions editor, Rob Calver, for his support and his patience throughout this book publishing project.

Frank Bretz, Torsten Hothorn and Peter Westfall
Basel, München and Lubbock

CHAPTER 1

Introduction

Many scientific experiments subject to rigorous statistical analyses involve the simultaneous evaluation of more than one question. For example, in clinical trials one may compare more than one treatment group with a control group, assess several outcome variables, measure at various time points, analyze multiple subgroups or look at any combination of these and related questions; but multiplicity problems occur if we want to make simultaneous inference across multiple questions. Similar problems may arise in agricultural field experiments which simultaneously compare several irrigation systems, investigate the dose response relationship of a fertilizer, involve repeated assessments of growth curves for a particular culture, etc. Recently, high-dimensional screening studies have become widely available in molecular biology and its applications, such as gene expression experiments and high throughput screenings in early drug discovery. Those screening studies have in common the problem of identifying a small subset of relevant variables from a huge set of candidate variables (e.g., genes, compounds, proteins). Scientific research provides many examples of well-designed experiments involving multiple investigational questions. Multiplicity is likely to become important when strong evidence and good decision making is required.

In hypotheses test problems involving a single null hypothesis H the statistical tests are often chosen to control the Type I error rate of incorrectly rejecting H at a pre-specified significance level α. If multiple hypotheses, m say, are tested simultaneously and the final inferences should be valid across all experimental questions of interest, the probability of declaring non-existing effects significant increases in m. Assume, for example, that $m = 2$ hypotheses H_1 and H_2 are each tested at level $\alpha = 0.05$ using independent test statistics. For example, let $H_i, i = 1, 2$, denote the null hypotheses that a drug does not show a beneficial effect over placebo for two primary outcome variables. Assume further that both H_1 and H_2 are true. Then the probability of retaining both hypotheses is $(1-\alpha)^2 = 0.9025$ under the independence assumption. The complementary probability of incorrectly rejecting at least one null hypothesis is $1 - (1 - \alpha)^2 = 2\alpha - \alpha^2 = 0.0975$. This is substantially larger than the initial significance level of $\alpha = 0.05$. In general, when testing m null hypotheses using independent test statistics, the probability of committing at least one Type I error is $1 - (1 - \alpha)^m$, which reduces to the previous expression for $m = 2$. Figure 1.1 displays the probability of committing at least one Type I error for $m = 1, \ldots, 100$ and $\alpha = 0.01, 0.05$, and 0.10. Clearly, the probability quickly reaches 1 for sufficiently large values of m. In other words, if there is a large number of experimental questions and no multiplicity adjustment, the decision maker will commit a Type I error almost surely and conclude for a seemingly significant effect when there is none.

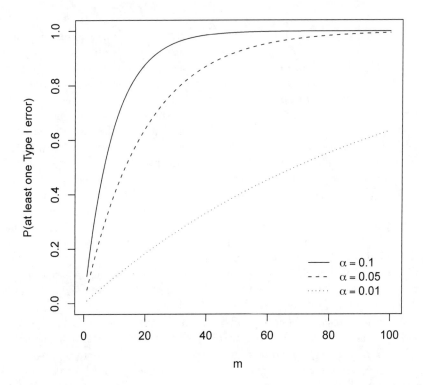

Figure 1.1   Probability of committing at least one Type I error for different significance levels α and number of hypotheses m.

To further illustrate the multiplicity issue, consider the problem of testing whether or not a given coin is fair. One may conclude that the coin was biased if after 10 flips the coin landed heads at least 9 times. Indeed, if one assumes as a null hypothesis that the coin is fair, then the likelihood that a fair coin would come up heads at least 9 out of 10 times is $11 \cdot (0.5)^{10} = 0.0107$. This is relatively unlikely, and under common statistical criteria such as whether the p-value is less than or equal to 0.05, one would reject the null hypothesis and conclude that the coin is unfair. While this approach may be appropriate for testing the fairness of a single coin, applying the same approach to test the fairness of many coins could lead to a multiplicity problem. Imagine if one was to test 100 fair coins by this method. Given that the probability of a fair coin coming up heads 9 or 10 times in 10 flips is 0.0107, one would expect that in flipping 100 fair coins 10 times each, it would still be very unlikely to see a particular (i.e., pre-specified) coin come up heads 9 or 10 times. However, it is more likely than not that at least one coin will behave this way, no matter which one. To be more precise, the likelihood that all 100 fair coins are identified as fair by this criterion is only $(1 - 0.0107)^{100} = 0.34$. In other words, the likelihood of declaring at least one of the 100 fair coins as unfair is 0.66; this result can also be approximated from Figure 1.1. Therefore, the application of our single-test coin-fairness criterion to multiple comparisons would more likely than not lead to a false conclusion: We would mistakenly identify a fair coin as unfair.

Let us consider a real data example to illustrate yet a different perspective of the multiplicity problem. Consider the `thuesen` regression example from Altman (1991) and reanalyzed by Dalgaard (2002). The data are available from the **ISwR** package (Dalgaard 2010) and contain the ventricular shortening velocity and blood glucose measurements for 23 Type I diabetic patients with complete observations. In Figure 1.2 we show a scatter plot of the data including the regression line. Assume that we are interested in fitting a linear regression model and subsequently in testing whether the intercept or the slope equal 0, resulting in two null hypotheses of interest. We will consider this example in more detail in Chapter 3, but we use it here to illustrate some of the multiplicity issues and how to address them in R.

Consider the linear model fit

```
R> thuesen.lm <- lm(short.velocity ~ blood.glucose,
+                   data = thuesen)
R> summary(thuesen.lm)

Call:
lm(formula = short.velocity ~ blood.glucose,
   data = thuesen)

Residuals:
   Min      1Q Median      3Q     Max
-0.401  -0.148 -0.022   0.030   0.435

Coefficients:
             Estimate Std. Error t value Pr(>|t|)
(Intercept)    1.0978     0.1175    9.34  6.3e-09 ***
blood.glucose  0.0220     0.0105    2.10    0.048 *
---
Signif. codes:  0 '***' 0.001 '**' 0.01 '*' 0.05 '.' 0.1 ' ' 1

Residual standard error: 0.217 on 21 degrees of freedom
  (1 observation deleted due to missingness)
Multiple R-squared: 0.174,        Adjusted R-squared: 0.134
F-statistic: 4.41 on 1 and 21 DF,  p-value: 0.0479
```

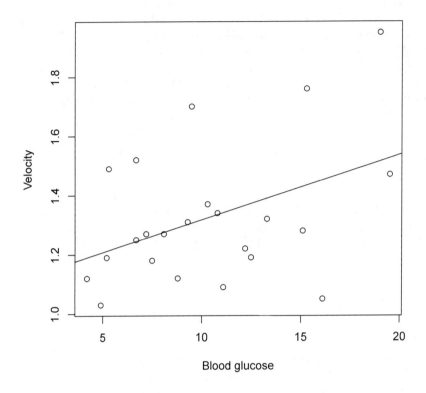

Figure 1.2   Scatter plot of the `thuesen` data with regression line.

From the p-values associated with the intercept ($p < 0.001$) and the slope ($p = 0.048$) one might be tempted to conclude that both parameters differ significantly from zero at the significance level $\alpha = 0.05$. However, these assessments are based on the *marginal* p-values, which do not account for a multiplicity adjustment. A better approach is to adjust the marginal p-values with a suitable multiple comparison procedure, such as the Bonferroni test. When applying the Bonferroni method, the marginal p-values are essentially multiplied by the number of null hypotheses to be tested (that is, by 2 in our example). One possibility to perform the Bonferroni test in R is to use the **multcomp** package. Understanding the details of the statements below will become clear when introducing the **multcomp** package formally in Chapter 3. For now we prefer to illustrate the key ideas without getting distracted by theoretical details.

```
R> library("multcomp")
R> thuesen.mc <- glht(thuesen.lm, linfct = diag(2))
R> summary(thuesen.mc, test = adjusted(type = "bonferroni"))
```

```
        Simultaneous Tests for General Linear Hypotheses

Fit: lm(formula = short.velocity ~ blood.glucose,
   data = thuesen)

Linear Hypotheses:
        Estimate Std. Error t value Pr(>|t|)
1 == 0    1.0978     0.1175    9.34  1.3e-08 ***
2 == 0    0.0220     0.0105    2.10    0.096 .
---
Signif. codes:  0 '***' 0.001 '**' 0.01 '*' 0.05 '.' 0.1 ' ' 1
(Adjusted p values reported -- bonferroni method)
```

In the column entitled Pr(>|t|), the slope parameter now fails to be significant. The associated adjusted p-value is 0.096, twice as large as the unadjusted p-value from the previous analysis. This is because now the p-value is corrected (i.e., adjusted) for multiplicity using the Bonferroni test. Thus, if the original aim was to draw a *simultaneous* inference across both experimental questions (that is, whether intercept or slope equal zero), one would conclude that the intercept is significantly different from 0 but the slope is not.

The **multcomp** package provides a variety of powerful improvements over the Bonferroni test. As a matter of fact, when calling the glht function above, the default approach accounts for the correlations between the parameter estimates. This leads to smaller p-values compared to the Bonferroni test, as shown in the output below:

```
R> summary(thuesen.mc)
```

```
        Simultaneous Tests for General Linear Hypotheses

Fit: lm(formula = short.velocity ~ blood.glucose,
   data = thuesen)

Linear Hypotheses:
        Estimate Std. Error t value Pr(>|t|)
1 == 0    1.0978     0.1175    9.34    1e-08 ***
2 == 0    0.0220     0.0105    2.10    0.064 .
---
Signif. codes:  0 '***' 0.001 '**' 0.01 '*' 0.05 '.' 0.1 ' ' 1
(Adjusted p values reported -- single-step method)
```

The adjusted p-value for the slope parameter is now 0.064 and thus considerably smaller than the 0.096 from the Bonferroni test, although we still have not achieved significance. During the course of this book we will discuss even more powerful methods, which allow the user to safely claim that the slope is significant at the level $\alpha = 0.05$ after having adjusted for multiplicity.

In summary, this example illustrates (i) the necessity of using proper multiple comparison procedures when aiming at simultaneous inference; (ii) a variety of different multiplicity adjustments, some of which are less powerful than others and should be avoided whenever possible; and (iii) the availability of flexible interfaces in R, such as the **multcomp** package, which provide fast results for data analysts interested in simultaneous inferences of multiple hypotheses.

We conclude this chapter with a few general considerations. Broadly speaking, multiplicity is a concern whenever reproducibility of results is required. That is, if an experiment needs to be repeated, not initially adjusting for multiplicity may increase the likelihood of observing different results in later experiments. Because scientific research and development can often be regarded as a sequence of experiments that confirm or add to the understanding of previously established results, reproducibility is an important aspect. According to Westfall and Bretz (2010), replication failure can happen in at least three ways. Assume that we are interested in assessing the effect of multiple conditions (treatments, genes, ...). It may then happen that

(i) a condition has an effect in the opposite direction than was reported in an experiment;

(ii) a condition has an effect, but one that is substantially smaller than was reported in an experiment;

(iii) a condition is ineffective, despite being reported as efficacious in an experiment.

Such failures to replicate are commonly attributed to flawed study designs and various types of biases; however, multiplicity is as likely a culprit. Further details about the three types of replication errors given above follow.

Errors of declaring effects in the "wrong direction". This is related to the problem of testing two-sided hypotheses with associated directional decisions. Although one might not believe point-zero null hypotheses can truly exist, two-sided tests are common and directional errors are real. It is likely that directions of the claims are erroneous when multiple comparisons are performed without multiplicity adjustment. For example, if a test of a two-sided hypothesis is done at the 0.05 level, then there is (at most) a 0.025 probability that the test will be declared significant, but in the wrong direction. When multiple tests are performed, this probability increases, so that if 40 tests are performed, we may expect one directional error (in a worst case). Note that although the probability of committing a directional error may be small, it has a severe impact once it is made because of the decision to the wrong direction.

Errors of declaring inflated effect sizes. A second characterization of the multiplicity problem is the impact on selection effects. In this scenario, we need not postulate directional errors. In fact, we may believe with a priori certainty that all effects are in their expected directions. Nevertheless, when we isolate a single, "most significant" comparison from this collection, we can only presume that the estimated effect size is biased upward due to selection effects.

Assume, for example, an experiment, where we investigate m treatments. If at the final analysis we select the "best" treatment based on the observed results, then the associated naïve treatment estimate will be biased upward. To illustrate this phenomenon, we assume that m random variables $x_1, \ldots, x_m$ associated with m distinct treatments are independently standard normally distributed. We consider selecting the treatment with the maximum observed value $\max\{x_1, \ldots, x_m\}$. Figure 1.3 displays the resulting density curves for different values of m. The shift in distribution towards larger values for increasing m is evident. In other words, if we would repeat an experiment a large number of times for $m = 5$ (say) treatment groups and at each time report the observed estimate for the selected treatment (that is, the one with the largest observed value), then the average reported estimate would be around 1 instead of 0 (which is the true value). The same pattern holds if the true effects are of equal size, but different from 0. Note that in practice the true bias may even be larger than suggested in Figure 1.3, if one were to only report the treatment effect estimates from successful experiments with statistically significant results. That is, in practice the selection bias observed in Figure 1.3 may be confounded with reporting bias (Bretz, Maurer, and Gallo 2009c). Finally, note from Figure 1.3 that multiplicity does not impact only the location of the distribution, but leads also to a reduction in the variability and an increase in the skewness as m increases.

Errors of declaring effects when none exist. The classical characterization of multiplicity is in terms of the "1 in 20" significance criterion: In 20 tests of hypotheses, all of which are (unknown to the analyst) truly null, we expect to commit one Type I error and incorrectly reject one of the 20 null hypotheses. Thus, *multiple testing* can increase the likelihood of Type I errors. This characterization is closely related to the motivating discussion at the beginning of this chapter and the probabilities displayed in Figure 1.1. In fact, much of the material in this book is devoted to this classical characterization and the description of suitable multiple comparison procedures, which account for the impact of multiple significance testing.

While we often attribute lack of replication to poor designs and data collection procedures, we should also consider selection effects related to multiplicity as a cause. In many cases these effects can be subtle. Consider, for example, a clinical efficacy measure taken one month after administration of a drug. The efficacy can be determined (a) using the raw measure, (b) using the percentage change from baseline, (c) using the actual change from baseline or (d) using the baseline covariate-adjusted raw measure. If we follow an aggressive strategy and chose the "best" (and most significant) measure, then the reported effect size measure will clearly be inflated, because the maximal statistic capitalizes (unfairly) on random variations in the data. In such a case, it is not surprising that follow-up studies may produce less stellar results; this phenomenon is an example of regression to the mean.

In all three characterizations above, there is a concern that the presentation of the scientific findings from an experiment may be exaggerated. In some areas

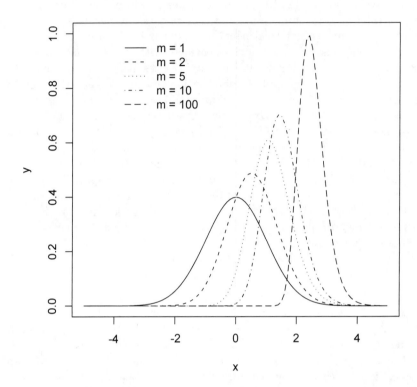

Figure 1.3   Density curves of the effect estimate after selecting the "best" treatment with the maximum observed response for different numbers m
of treatments.

(especially in the health care environment) regulatory agencies recognized this
problem and released corresponding (international) guidelines to ensure a good
statistical practice. In 1998, the International Conference on Harmonization
published a tripartite guideline for statistical principles in clinical trials (ICH
1998), which reflects concerns with multiplicity:

> When multiplicity is present, the usual frequentist approach to the analysis of
> clinical trial data may necessitate an adjustment to the Type I error. Multiplicity
> may arise, for example, from multiple primary variables, multiple comparisons of
> treatments, repeated evaluation over time, and/or interim analyses ... [multiplic-
> ity] adjustment should always be considered and the details of any adjustment
> procedure or an explanation of why adjustment is not thought to be necessary
> should be set out in the analysis plan.

In addition, the European Medicines Agency in its Committee for Proprietary

Medicinal Products document "Points to Consider on Multiplicity Issues in Clinical Trials" (EMEA 2002), states that

> ... multiplicity can have a substantial influence on the rate of false positive conclusions whenever there is an opportunity to choose the most favorable results from two or more analyses ...

and later echoes the ICH recommendation to state details of the multiple comparison procedure in the analysis plan. While these documents allow that multiplicity adjustment might not be necessary, they also request justifications for such action. As a result, pharmaceutical companies have routinely begun to incorporate adequate multiple comparison procedures in their statistical analyses. But even if guidelines are not available or do not apply, control of multiplicity is to the experimenter's advantage as it ensures better decision making and safeguards against selection bias.

CHAPTER 2

General Concepts and Basic Multiple Comparison Procedures

The objective of this chapter is to introduce general concepts related to multiple testing as well as to describe basic strategies for constructing multiple comparison procedures. In Section 2.1 we introduce relevant error rates used for multiple hypotheses test problems. In addition, we discuss general concepts, such as adjusted and unadjusted p-values, single-step and stepwise test procedures, etc. In Section 2.2 we review different principles of constructing multiple comparison procedures, including union-intersection tests, intersection-union tests, the closure principle and the partitioning principle. We then review commonly used multiple comparison procedures constructed from marginal p-values. Methods presented here include Bonferroni-type methods and their improvements (Section 2.3) as well as modified Bonferroni methods based on the Simes inequality (Section 2.4). For each method, we describe its assumptions, advantages and limitations.

2.1 Error rates and general concepts

In this section we introduce relevant error rates for multiple comparison procedures, which extend the familiar error rates used when testing a single null hypothesis. We also introduce general concepts important to multiple hypotheses testing, including weak and strong error rate control, adjusted and unadjusted p-values, single-step and stepwise test procedures, simultaneous confidence intervals, coherence, consonance and the properties of free and restricted combinations. For more detailed discussions of these and related topics we refer the reader to the books by Hochberg and Tamhane (1987) and Hsu (1996) as well as to the articles on general multiple test methodology by Lehmann (1957a,b); Gabriel (1969); Marcus, Peritz, and Gabriel (1976); Sonnemann (1982); Stefansson, Kim, and Hsu (1988); Finner and Strassburger (2002) and the references therein.

2.1.1 Error rates

Type I error rates

Let $m \geq 1$ denote the number of null hypotheses $H_1, \ldots, H_m$ to be tested. Assume each *elementary hypothesis* $H_i, i = 1, \ldots, m$, is associated with a given experimental question of interest. The number m of null hypotheses is application specific and can vary substantially from one case to another. For example, standard clinical dose finding studies compare a small number of distinct dose levels of a new drug, $m = 4$ say, with a control treatment. The elementary hypothesis H_i then states that the treatment effect at dose level i is not better than the effect under the control, $i = 1, \ldots, 4$. The number m of hypotheses can be in the 1,000s in a microarray experiment, where a null hypothesis H_i may state that gene i is not differentially expressed under two comparative conditions (Dudoit and van der Laan 2008). Finally, the number of hypotheses is infinite when constructing simultaneous confidence bands over a continuous covariate region (Liu 2010).

For any test problem, there are three types of errors. A false positive decision occurs if we declare an effect when none exists. Similarly, a false negative decision occurs if we fail to declare a truly existing effect. In hypotheses test problems, these errors are denoted as Type I and Type II errors, respectively. The correct rejection of a null hypothesis coupled with a wrong directional decision is denoted as Type III error. The related notation is summarized in Table 2.1. Let $M = \{1, \ldots, m\}$ denote the index set associated with the null hypotheses $H_1, \ldots, H_m$ and let $M_0 \subseteq M$ denote the set of $m_0 = |M_0|$ true hypotheses, where $|A|$ denotes the cardinality of a set A. In Table 2.1, V denotes the number of Type I errors and R the number of rejected hypotheses. Note that R is an observable random variable, S, T, U, and V are all unobservable random variables, while m and m_0 are fixed numbers, where m_0 is unknown.

Hypotheses	Not Rejected	Rejected	Total
True	U	V	m_0
False	T	S	$m - m_0$
Total	W	R	m

Table 2.1   Type I and II errors in multiple hypotheses testing.

A standard approach in univariate hypothesis testing ($m = 1$) is to choose an appropriate test, which maintains the Type I error rate at a pre-specified significance level α. Different extensions of the univariate Type I error rate to multiple test problems are possible. In the following we review several error rate definitions commonly used for multiple comparison procedures.

The *per-comparison error rate*

$$\text{PCER} = \frac{\mathbb{E}(V)}{m}$$

is the expected proportion of Type I errors among the m decisions. If each of the m hypotheses is tested separately at a pre-specified significance level α, then $\text{PCER} = \alpha m_0 / m \leq \alpha$.

In many applications, however, controlling the per-comparison error rate at level α is not considered adequate. Instead, the hypotheses $H_1, \ldots, H_m$ are considered jointly as a family, where a single Type I error already leads to an incorrect decision. This motivates the use of the *familywise error rate*

$$\text{FWER} = \mathbb{P}(V > 0),$$

which is the probability of committing at least one Type I error. The familywise error rate is the most common error rate used in multiple testing, particularly historically, and also in current practice where the number of comparisons is moderate and/or where strong evidence is needed. The familywise error rate is closely related to the motivating considerations from Chapter 1. From Figure 1.1 we can see that FWER approaches 1 for moderate to large number of hypotheses m if there is no multiplicity adjustment. Note that the familywise error rate reduces to the common Type I error rate for $m = 1$.

When the number m of hypotheses is very large and/or when strong evidence is not required (as is typically the case in high-dimensional screening studies in molecular biology or early drug discovery), control of the familywise error rate can be too strict. That is, if the probability of missing differential effects is too high, the use of the familywise error rate may not be appropriate. In this case, a straightforward extension of the familywise error rate is to consider the probability of committing more than k Type I errors for a pre-specified number k: If the total number of hypotheses m is large, a small number k of Type I errors may be acceptable. This leads to the *generalized familywise error rate* $\text{gFWER} = \mathbb{P}(V > k)$, see Victor (1982); Hommel and Hoffmann (1988), and Lehmann and Romano (2005) for details. Control of the generalized familywise error rate is less stringent than control of the familywise error rate at a common significance level α: A method controlling the generalized familywise error rate may allow, with high probability, a few Type I errors, provided that the number is less than or equal to the pre-specified number k. On the other hand, methods controlling the familywise error rate ensure that the probability of committing *any* Type I error is bounded by α.

An alternative approach is to relate the number V of false positives to the total number R of rejections. Let $Q = V/R$ if $R > 0$ and $Q = 0$ otherwise. The *false discovery rate*

$$
\begin{aligned}
\text{FDR} &= \mathbb{E}(Q) \\
&= \mathbb{E}\left(\frac{V}{R} \,\middle|\, R > 0\right) \mathbb{P}(R > 0) + 0 \cdot \mathbb{P}(R = 0) \\
&= \mathbb{E}\left(\frac{V}{R} \,\middle|\, R > 0\right) \mathbb{P}(R > 0)
\end{aligned}
$$

is then the expected proportion of falsely rejected hypotheses among the rejected hypotheses (Benjamini and Hochberg 1995). Earlier ideas related to the false discovery rate can be found in Seeger (1968) and Sorić (1989). The introduction of the false discovery rate has initiated the investigation of alternative error control criteria and many further measures have been proposed recently. Storey (2003), for example, proposed the *positive false discovery rate pFDR =*

$\mathbb{E}(V/R|R > 0)$, which is defined as the expected proportion of falsely rejected hypotheses among the rejected hypotheses given that some are rejected. A different concept is to control the proportion V/R directly: Korn, Troendle, McShane, and Simon (2004) and van der Laan, Dudoit, and Pollard (2004) independently introduced computer-intensive multiple comparison procedures to control the *proportion of false positives* $PFP = \mathbb{P}(V/R > g), 0 < g < 1$. For a recent review we refer the reader to Benjamini (2010) and the references therein.

In general,

$$\text{PCER} \leq \text{FDR} \leq \text{FWER}$$

for a given multiple comparison procedure. This can be seen by noting that $V/m \leq Q \leq \mathbf{1}_{\{V>0\}}$, where the indicator function $\mathbf{1}_A = 1$ if an event A is true and $\mathbf{1}_A = 0$ otherwise, and that $\text{PCER} = \mathbb{E}(V/m)$, $\text{FDR} = \mathbb{E}(Q)$, and $\text{FWER} = \mathbb{E}(\mathbf{1}_{\{V>0\}})$. Thus, a multiple comparison procedure which controls the familywise error rate also controls the false discovery rate and the per-comparison error rate, but not vice versa. In contrast, familywise error rate controlling procedures are more conservative than false discovery rate controlling procedures in the sense that they lead to a smaller number of rejected hypotheses. In any case, good scientific practice requires the specification of the Type I error rate control to be done prior to the data analysis.

For any of the error concepts above, the error control is denoted as *weak*, if the Type I error rate is controlled only under the *global null hypothesis*

$$H = \bigcap_{i \in M_0} H_i, \quad M_0 = M,$$

which assumes that all null hypotheses $H_1, \ldots, H_m$ are true. Consequently, in case of controlling the familywise error rate in the weak sense, it is required that

$$\mathbb{P}(V > 0|H) \leq \alpha.$$

Consider an experiment investigating a new treatment for multiple outcome variables. Controlling the familywise error rate in the weak sense then implies the control of the probability of declaring an effect for at least one outcome variable, when there is no effect on any variable. In practice, however, it is unlikely that all null hypotheses are true and the global null hypothesis H is rarely expected to hold. Thus, a stronger error rate control under less restrictive assumptions is often necessary. If, for a given multiple comparison procedure, the Type I error rate is controlled under any partial configuration of true and false null hypotheses, the error control is denoted as *strong*. For example, to control the familywise error rate strongly it is required that

$$\max_{I \subseteq M} \mathbb{P}\left(V > 0 \,\Big|\, \bigcap_{i \in I} H_i\right) \leq \alpha,$$

where the maximum is taken over all possible configurations $\emptyset \neq I \subseteq M$ of true null hypotheses. In the previous example, controlling the familywise error rate in the strong sense implies the control of the probability of declaring an effect for at least one outcome variable, regardless of the effect sizes for any of the outcome variables. Note that if $m_0 = 0$, then $V = 0$ and FDR $= 0$. If $m_0 = m$, then FDR $= \mathbb{E}(1|R > 0)\mathbb{P}(R > 0) = \mathbb{P}(R > 0) = $ FWER. Hence, any false discovery rate controlling multiple comparison procedure also controls the familywise error rate in the weak sense.

Having introduced different measures for Type I errors in multiple test problems, we are now able to formally define a *multiple comparison procedure* as any statistical test procedure designed to account for and properly control the multiplicity effect through a suitable error rate. In this book, we focus on applications where the number of comparisons is moderate and/or where strong evidence is needed. Thus, we restrict our attention to multiple comparison procedures controlling the familywise error rate in the strong sense.

The appropriate choice of null hypotheses being of primary interest is a controversial question. That is, it is not always clear which set of hypotheses should constitute the family $H_1, \ldots, H_m$. This topic has often been in dispute and there is no general consensus. Any solution will necessarily be application specific and at its best serve as an example for other areas. Westfall and Bretz (2010), for example, provided some guidance, on when and how to adjust for multiplicity at different stages of drug development.

Type II error rates

A common requirement for any statistical test is to maximize the power and thereby to minimize the Type II error rate for a given Type I error criterion. Power considerations are thus an integral part of designing a scientific experiment. Analogous to extending the Type I error rate, power can be generalized in various ways when moving from single to multiple hypotheses test problems. Power concepts to measure an experiment's success are then associated with the probability of rejecting an elementary null hypothesis $H_i, i \in M$, when in fact H_i is not true. The problem is that the individual events

$$\text{``}H_i \text{ is rejected''} , \quad i \in M,$$

can be combined in different ways, thus leading to different measures of success. Below we use the notation from Table 2.1 to briefly review some common power concepts.

The *individual power*

$$\pi_i^{\text{ind}} = \mathbb{P}(\text{reject } H_i), \quad i \in M_1 = M \setminus M_0,$$

is the rejection probability for a false hypothesis H_i. The concept of *average power* is closely related to individual power. It is defined as the average expected number of correct rejections among all false null hypotheses, that is,

$$\pi^{\text{ave}} = \frac{\mathbb{E}(S)}{m_1} = \frac{1}{m_1} \sum_{i \in M_1} \pi_i^{\text{ind}},$$

where $m_1 = |M_1|$ denotes the number of false null hypotheses. Alternatively, the *disjunctive power*

$$\pi^{\text{dis}} = \mathbb{P}(S \geq 1)$$

is the probability of rejecting at least one false null hypothesis. An appealing feature of the disjunctive power is that π^{dis} decreases to the familywise error rate as the effect sizes related to the false null hypotheses $H_i, i \in M_1$, decrease. In contrast, the *conjunctive power*

$$\pi^{\text{con}} = \mathbb{P}(S = m_1)$$

is the probability of rejecting all false null hypotheses. Note that disjunctive and conjunctive power have also been referred to as multiple (or minimal) and total (or complete) power, respectively; see Maurer and Mellein (1988) and Westfall et al. (1999). But since $\pi^{\text{dis}} \geq \pi^{\text{con}}$, these naming conventions often lead to confusion (Senn and Bretz 2007). When the family of tests consists of pairwise mean comparisons, the previously mentioned power measures have been introduced as per-pair power, any-pair power, and all-pairs power (Ramsey 1978). Finally, it should be noted that these power definitions are readily extended to any subset $M_1' \subseteq M_1$ of false null hypotheses. Note also that all of these probabilities are conditional on which null hypotheses are true and which are false.

The relevant practical question is to determine the appropriate power concept to use for a given study. One may argue that conjunctive power should be used in studies that aim at detecting all existing effects, such as in intersection union settings, see Section 2.2.2. Disjunctive power is recommended in studies that aim at detecting at least one true effect, such as in union intersection settings, see Section 2.2.1. Individual power is appealing in clinical trials with multiple secondary outcome variables (Bretz, Maurer, and Hommel 2010) and average power can be useful for comparing different multiple comparison procedures. In general, however, a suitable power definition can be given only on a case-by-case basis by choosing power measures tailored to the study objectives.

Directional errors

A particular issue arises in two-sided test problems, when the elementary hypotheses $H_1, \ldots, H_m$ are point-null hypotheses. Having rejected H_i, the natural inclination is to make a directional decision on the sign of the effect being tested. This requires control of both Type I errors and errors in determining the sign of non-null effects. A *directional error* (also known as Type III error) is defined as the rejection of a false null hypotheses, where the sign of the true effect parameter is opposite to the one of its sample estimate.

Let A_1 denote the event of at least one Type I error such that $\mathbb{P}(A_1) = $ FWER. Let further A_2 denote the event that there is at least one sign error among the true non-null effects. The problem becomes how to control the *combined error rate* $\mathbb{P}(A_1 \cup A_2)$ at a pre-specified level. Stepwise test procedures (see Section 2.1.2 for a definition) are powerful methods for controlling the familywise error rate, but do not necessarily control the combined error rate.

Shaffer (1980) gave a counterexample involving shifted Cauchy distributions; however, she also noted that for independent test statistics satisfying certain distributional conditions (which include the normal but rule out the Cauchy case), the combined error rate is controlled by the Holm procedure from Section 2.3.2 (Holm 1979a). Moreover, Holm (1979b) noted the control of the combined error rate for conditionally independent tests including noncentral multivariate t with identity dispersion matrix. Finner (1999) further extended the class of stepwise tests that control the combined error rate to include some step-up tests, closed F tests, and modified S method tests. He also noted that while specialized procedures guaranteeing combined error rate control have been developed (see, for example, Bauer, Hackl, Hommel, and Sonnemann (1986)), they are often less powerful than standard closed and stepwise tests. Westfall, Tobias, and Bretz (2000) systematically investigated combined error rates of stepwise test procedures relevant to analysis-of-variance models involving correlated comparisons, using both analytic and simulation-based methods. No cases of excess directional error were found for typical applications involving noncentral multivariate t distributions.

2.1.2 General concepts

Single-step and stepwise procedures

One possibility of classifying multiple comparison procedures is to divide them into single-step and stepwise procedures. *Single-step procedures* are characterized by the fact that the rejection or non-rejection of a null hypothesis does not take the decision for any other hypothesis into account. Thus, the order in which the hypotheses are tested is not important and one can think of the multiple inferences as being performed in a single step. A well-known example of a single-step procedure is the Bonferroni test. In contrast, for *stepwise procedures* the rejection or non-rejection of a null hypothesis may depend on the decision of other hypotheses. The equally well-known Holm procedure is a stepwise extension of the Bonferroni test using the closure principle under the free combination condition (see Section 2.3 for a description of these procedures).

Stepwise procedures are further divided into step-down and step-up procedures. Both types of procedures assume a sequence of hypotheses $H_1 \prec \ldots \prec H_m$, where the ordering "$\prec$" of the hypotheses can be data dependent. *Step-down procedures* start testing the first ordered hypothesis H_1 and step down through the sequence while rejecting the hypotheses. The procedure stops at the first non-rejection (at H_i, say), and $H_1, \ldots, H_{i-1}$ are rejected. The Holm procedure is an example of a step-down procedure. *Step-up procedures* start testing H_m and step up through the sequence while retaining the hypotheses. The procedure stops at the first rejection (at H_i, say), and $H_1, \ldots, H_i$ are all rejected.

Single-step procedures are generally less powerful than their stepwise extensions in the sense that any hypothesis rejected by the former will also be

rejected by the latter, but not vice versa. This will become clear when introducing the closure principle in Section 2.2.3. The power advantage of stepwise
test procedures, however, comes at the cost of increased difficulties in constructing compatible simultaneous confidence intervals for the parameter of
interest, which have a joint coverage probability of at least $1 - \alpha$ (see below).

Adjusted p-values

The computation of p-values is a common exercise in univariate hypothesis
test problems. Therefore, it is desirable to also compute *adjusted p-values*
for a given multiple comparison procedure, which are directly comparable
with the significance level α. An adjusted p-value q_i is defined as the smallest
significance level for which one still rejects the elementary hypothesis $H_i, i \in$
M, given a particular multiple comparison procedure. In case of the familywise
error rate,

$$q_i = \inf\{\alpha \in (0,1)|H_i \text{ is rejected at level } \alpha\},$$

if such an α exists, and $q_i = 1$ otherwise; see Westfall and Young (1993)
and Wright (1992). Adjusted p-values capture by construction the multiplicity adjustment induced through a given multiple comparison procedure and
incorporate the potentially complex underlying decision rules. Consequently,
whenever $q_i \leq \alpha$, the associated elementary null hypothesis H_i can be rejected
while controlling the familywise error rate at level α. Examples of computing
adjusted p-values are given later when we describe the individual multiple
comparison procedures. The marginal p-values p_i are denoted as *unadjusted
p-values* in this book.

Simultaneous confidence intervals

The duality between testing and confidence intervals is well established in
univariate hypotheses test problems (Lehmann 1986). A general method for
constructing a confidence set from a significance test is as follows. Let θ denote the parameter of interest. For each parameter point θ_0, test the hypothesis
$H: \theta = \theta_0$ at level α. The set of all parameter points θ_0, for which $H: \theta = \theta_0$
is accepted, constitutes a confidence set for the true value of θ with coverage
probability $1 - \alpha$. This method is essentially based on partitioning the parameter space into subsets, where each subset consists of a single parameter
point.

The partitioning principle described in Section 2.2.4 provides a natural extension for deriving compatible simultaneous confidence intervals in multiple
test problems, which have a joint coverage probability of at least $1 - \alpha$ for the
parameters of interest (Finner and Strassburger 2002). Here, compatibility between a multiple comparison procedure and a set of simultaneous confidence
intervals means that if a null hypothesis is rejected with the test procedure,
then the associated multiplicity corrected confidence interval excludes all parameter values for which the null hypothesis is true (Hayter and Hsu 1994).

Applying the partitioning principle, the parameter space is partitioned into small disjoint subhypotheses, where each is tested appropriately. The union of all non-rejected hypotheses then yields a confidence set C for the parameter vector of interest. Note that the finest possible partition is given by a pointwise partition such that each point of the parameter space represents an element of the partition. Most of the classical (simultaneous) confidence intervals can be derived by using the finest partition and an appropriate family of one- or two-sided tests. In general, however, this may not be the case, although a confidence set C can always be used to construct simultaneous confidence intervals by simply projecting C on the coordinate axes. Compatibility can be ensured by enforcing mild conditions on the partition and the test family (Strassburger, Bretz, and Hochberg 2004).

Simultaneous confidence intervals are available in closed form for many standard single-step procedures and will be used in Chapters 3 and 4. Simultaneous confidence intervals for stepwise procedures, however, are usually more difficult to derive and often have limited practical use. We refer to Strassburger and Bretz (2008) and Guilbaud (2008, 2009) for recent results and discussions.

Free and restricted combinations

A family of null hypotheses $H_i, i \in M$, satisfies the *free combination* condition if for any subset $I \subseteq M$ the simultaneous truth of $H_i, i \in I$, and falsehood of the remaining hypotheses is a plausible event. Otherwise, the hypotheses $H_1, \ldots, H_m$ satisfy the *restricted combination* condition (Holm 1979a; Westfall and Young 1993).

As an example of a hypotheses family satisfying the free combination condition, consider the comparison of two treatments with a control treatment (resulting in $m = 2$ null hypotheses). Any of the three events "none/one/both of the treatments is better than the control treatment" is then a plausible configuration and likely to be true in practice. As an example of a hypotheses family satisfying the restricted combination condition, consider all pairwise comparisons of three treatments means θ_1, θ_2, and θ_3 (resulting in $m = 3$ null hypotheses). In this example, not all configurations of null and alternative hypotheses are logically possible. For example, if $\theta_1 \neq \theta_2$, then $\theta_1 = \theta_3$ and $\theta_2 = \theta_3$ cannot be true simultaneously, thus restricting the possible configurations of true and false null hypotheses.

The motivation for the distinction between free and restricted combinations will become clear later when deriving stepwise test procedures based on the closure principle. The Holm procedure (Section 2.3.2) and the step-down Dunnett procedure (Section 4.1.2) are both examples of a large class of closed test procedures tailored to hypotheses satisfying the free combination condition. Correspondingly, the Shaffer procedure (Section 2.3.2) and the closed Tukey test (Section 4.2.2) are examples of closed test procedures for restricted hypotheses.

Coherence and consonance

A multiple comparison procedure is called *coherent* if it has the following property: If $H_i \subseteq H_j$ and H_j is rejected, then H_i is rejected as well (Gabriel 1969). Coherence is an important requirement for any multiple comparison procedure. If coherence is not satisfied, problems with the interpretation of the test results may occur. The closed test procedures described in Section 2.2.3 are coherent by construction. By contrast, the Holm procedure described in Section 2.3.2 is coherent with free combinations, but in special cases involving restricted combinations, may not be coherent (Hommel and Bretz 2008). Note that any non-coherent multiple comparison procedure can be replaced by a coherent procedure which is uniformly at least as powerful (Sonnemann and Finner 1988).

Consonance is another desirable property of multiple comparison procedures, although it is not as important as coherence. Let $H_I = \bigcap_{i \in I} H_i$ denote the intersection hypothesis for an index set $I \subseteq M$. Furthermore, denote a hypothesis H_I as non-maximal if there is at least one $J \subseteq M$ with $H_J \supsetneq H_I$; otherwise, denote H_I as as maximal. Consonance implies that if a non-maximal hypothesis H_I is rejected, one can reject at least one maximal hypothesis $H_J \supseteq H_I$ (Gabriel 1969). In many applications, the elementary null hypotheses $H_1, \ldots, H_m$ are maximal. Consonance then ensures that if an intersection hypothesis H_I is rejected, at least one elementary hypothesis H_i with $i \in I$ can be rejected as well. Consonance will become important later when describing max-t tests that allow one to draw inferences about the individual null hypotheses H_i (Section 2.2.1), and it will become the basis to construct efficient shortcut procedures (Section 2.2.3). A more rigorous discussion of consonance can be found in Brannath and Bretz (2010).

2.2 Construction methods for multiple comparison procedures

We now consider different methods to construct multiple comparison procedures. These include union intersection (and intersection union) tests to construct multiple comparison procedures for the intersection (union) of several elementary null hypotheses. The closure principle and the recently introduced partitioning principle are powerful tools, which extend the union intersection test principle to obtain individual assessments for the elementary null hypotheses.

2.2.1 Union intersection test

Historically, the union intersection test was the first construction method for multiple comparison procedures (Roy 1953; Roy and Bose 1953). Assume, for example, that several irrigation systems are compared with a control. It is natural to claim success if at least one of the comparative irrigation systems leads to better results than the control. If H_i denotes the elementary hypoth-

esis of no difference in effect between irrigation system i and control, we wish
to correctly reject any (but at least one) false H_i.

To formalize this multiple comparison problem, consider a family of null
hypotheses H_i with associated alternative hypotheses $K_i, i \in M$. We are then
interested in testing the intersection null hypothesis $H = \bigcap_{i \in M} H_i$. One approach is to use test statistics $t_i, i \in M$, and reject H if any t_i exceeds its
associated critical value c_i. The rejection region is thus a union of rejection
regions, $\bigcup_{i \in M} \{t_i > c_i\}$, giving rise to the "union" in the "union intersection"
term. In summary, this construction leads to *union intersection tests*, which
test the intersection of the null hypotheses H_i against the union of the alternative hypotheses K_i, that is,

$$H = \bigcap_{i \in M} H_i \quad \text{against} \quad K = \bigcup_{i \in M} K_i.$$

Note that union intersection tests consider the global intersection null hypothesis H without formally allowing individual assessments of the elementary
hypotheses $H_1, \ldots, H_m$. That is, if H is rejected by a union intersection test,
one is still left with the question, which of the elementary hypotheses H_i
should be rejected. This shortcoming can be dealt with in numerous ways,
including simultaneous confidence interval construction in Section 2.1.2, or by
applying the closure principle described in Section 2.2.3. It turns out that the
union intersection test procedure dovetails nicely with multiple comparison
procedures in general; many of the procedures described in this book take the
union intersection method as a foundation.

Max-t tests form an important class of union intersection tests and will
become essential in Chapters 3 and 4. Let $t_1, \ldots, t_m$ denote the individual
test statistics associated with the hypotheses $H_1, \ldots, H_m$. Assume without
loss of generality that larger values of t_i favor the rejection of H_i. A natural
approach is then to consider the maximum of the individual test statistics t_i,
leading to the max-t test

$$t_{\max} = \max\{t_1, \ldots, t_m\}. \tag{2.1}$$

We then reject the global null hypothesis H if and only if $t_{\max} \geq c$, where
the common constant c is chosen to control the Type I error rate at level
α, that is, $\mathbb{P}(t_{\max} \geq c | H) = \alpha$. The critical value c is calculated from the
joint distribution of the random variables $t_1, \ldots, t_m$. Determining c is often
difficult or sometimes even impossible if that joint distribution is not available
or numerically intractable, and conservative solutions have to be applied.

It follows from Gabriel (1969) that applying max-t tests often leads to coherent and consonant multiple comparison procedures, giving rise to their
practical importance. Many popular multiple comparison procedures are in
fact max-t tests by construction, such as the Bonferroni test (Section 2.3.1),
the Dunnett test (Section 4.1.1), or the Tukey test (Section 4.2.1). In addition, powerful stepwise test procedures can be derived based on the closure

principle, which allows us to assess the elementary hypotheses $H_1, \ldots, H_m$ (Hochberg and Tamhane 1987, p. 55); see Section 2.2.3 for further details.

Note that if smaller values of t_i favor the rejection of H_i, the minimum of the individual test statistics t_i has to be taken instead. Because this is conceptually similar to Equation (2.1), we use the common term max-t tests, regardless of the sideness of the test problem. In two-sided test problems the maximum is taken over the absolute values of the individual test statistics, that is, $t_{\max} = \max\{|t_1|, \ldots, |t_m|\}$. Finally, note that the individual test statistics t_i (or, equivalently, their associated p-values p_i) can be combined in other ways instead of taking their maximum; see Westfall (2005) for an overview.

2.2.2 Intersection union test

Consider the following example from drug development. International guidelines require that combination therapies (that is, the simultaneous administration of two or more medications) have to show a clinical benefit against all individual monotherapies before being considered for market release (EMEA 2009). In contrast to the union intersection settings considered in Section 2.2.1, here it is required that all null hypotheses of no beneficial effect are rejected in order to claim that the combination therapy has a beneficial effect.

Formally, we are given the test problem

$$H' = \bigcup_{i \in M} H_i \quad \text{versus} \quad K' = \bigcap_{i \in M} K_i.$$

The *intersection union test* then rejects the union null hypothesis H' at overall level α, if all elementary hypothesis H_i are rejected by their local α-level tests (Berger 1982). If all test statistics $t_i, i \in M$, have the same marginal distribution, the intersection union test rejects H' if and only if $\min_{i \in M} t_i \geq c$, where c is the $(1 - \alpha)$-quantile from that marginal distribution. In this particular case the intersection union test is also known as *min-test*, as coined by Laska and Meisner (1989). Suppose that in the example above we have t test statistics comparing the combination therapy with the individual monotherapies. The hypothesis H' is rejected and we conclude for a beneficial effect of the combination therapy, if the smallest t test statistic is larger than the $(1 - \alpha)$-quantile from the univariate t distribution.

Note that if only some of the null hypotheses H_i are rejected locally (for example, $t_i > c$ for some i in case of the min-test), the union null hypothesis H' is retained and no individual assessments are possible. In such cases no elementary null hypothesis H_i can be rejected, because otherwise the family-wise error rate may not be controlled. This property often leads to the misconception that the intersection union test is conservative in the sense that the nominal Type I error rate is not exhausted and therefore the test would lack in power. In fact, the intersection union test fully exploits the Type I error and is moreover uniformly most powerful within a certain class of monotone α-level tests (Laska and Meisner 1989). Improvements, which discard the monotonicity condition or restrict the parameter space, can be found in Sarkar, Snapinn, and Wang (1995) and Patel (1991), respectively. Compatible confidence intervals for intersection union tests involving two hypotheses are given by Strassburger et al. (2004).

2.2.3 Closure principle

The union intersection tests from Section 2.2.1 test the global null hypothesis H without formally assessing the individual hypotheses $H_1, \ldots, H_m$. That is, if $H = \bigcap_{i \in M} H_i$ is rejected by a union intersection test, we cannot make any conclusions about the elementary hypotheses H_i. The *closure principle* introduced by Marcus et al. (1976) is a general construction method which leads to stepwise test procedures (Section 2.1.2) and allows one to draw individual conclusions about the elementary hypotheses H_i.

To describe the closure principle, we consider initially the case of $m = 2$ null hypotheses H_1 and H_2 and discuss the general case later. Suppose we want to assess whether any of two treatments (for example, two new drugs or irrigations systems) is better than a control treatment. Let μ_j denote the mean effect for treatment j, where $j = 0$ (control), $1, 2$. Let further $\theta_i = \mu_i - \mu_0$ denote the mean effect difference between treatment $i = 1, 2$ and the control. The θ_i are the parameters of interest and the resulting elementary null hypotheses are $H_i: \theta_i \leq 0, i = 1, 2$. When using the Bonferroni test (which is formally described in Section 2.3), each hypothesis H_i is tested at level $\alpha/2$ in order to control the familywise error rate at level α. However, the Bonferroni test can be improved by applying the closure principle, as described now.

It is useful to formally consider the hypotheses H_i as subsets of the parameter space, about which we want to draw our inferences. Let $\Theta = \mathbb{R}^2$ denote the parameter space with $\boldsymbol{\theta} = (\theta_1, \theta_2) \in \Theta$. Figure 2.1 visualizes the hypotheses $H_i = \{\boldsymbol{\theta} \in \mathbb{R}^2 : \theta_i \leq 0\}$, $i = 1, 2$, as subsets of the real plane (the parameter space). Clearly, the two elementary hypotheses H_1 and H_2 are not disjoint: The intersection of both is given by $H_{12} = H_1 \cap H_2 = \{\boldsymbol{\theta} \in \mathbb{R}^2 : \theta_1 \leq 0 \text{ and } \theta_2 \leq 0\}$, which is the lower left quadrant in Figure 2.1. Testing the intersection hypothesis H_{12} requires an adjustment for multiplicity. This is taken into account by the Bonferroni test, which actually tests the entire union $H_1 \cup H_2$ at level $\alpha/2$ and not just the intersection hypothesis H_{12}. However, Figure 2.1 suggests that the remaining parts $H_1 \setminus H_{12}$ and $H_2 \setminus H_{12}$ can each be tested at full level α, without the need to adjust further for multiplicity. This leads to the "natural" test strategy of first testing the intersection hypothesis H_{12} with an appropriate union intersection test, and, if this is significant, continue testing H_1 and H_2, each at full level α. The null hypothesis H_1 is rejected (while controlling the familywise error rate strongly at level α) if and only if both H_1 and H_{12} are rejected, each at (local) level α. Conversely, H_2 is rejected if both H_2 and H_{12} are rejected. If H_{12} is not rejected at first place, further testing is unnecessary; otherwise, if H_1 (say) is rejected, but H_{12} is not, this would lead to interpretation problems (coherence property, see Section 2.1.2). This construction method is the key idea of the closure principle.

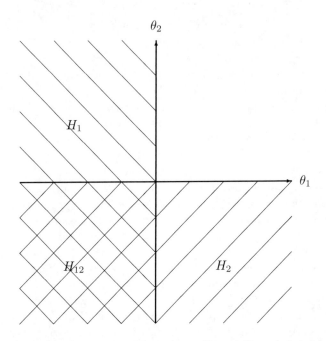

Figure 2.1   Visualization of two null hypotheses H_1 and H_2 and their intersection H_{12} in the parameter space $\mathbb{R}^2$.

There are alternative possibilities of visualizing the closure principle than shown in Figure 2.1. In Figure 2.2 we provide a Venn-type diagram for two null hypotheses H_1 and H_2 and their intersection H_{12}. In Figure 2.3 we show a related schematic diagram, which provides a convenient way of visualizing the test dependencies among the hypotheses. The intersection hypothesis H_{12} is shown at the top, while the two elementary hypotheses H_1 and H_2 are shown at the bottom of the diagram. Testing occurs in a "top-down" fashion. As described above, H_{12} is tested with a union intersection test at level α. If H_{12} is not rejected, further testing is unnecessary. Otherwise, H_1 and H_2 are each tested at level α. Finally, H_1 is rejected (while controlling the familywise error rate strongly at level α) if H_{12} and H_1 are both locally rejected. A similar decision rule holds also for H_2.

We now consider the case of testing any number m of null hypotheses $H_i, i = 1, \ldots, m$ (such as comparing m treatments with a control). The closure principle considers all intersection hypotheses constructed from the initial hypotheses set. Each intersection hypothesis is tested at local level α. Note that we can specify any α-level union intersection test for the intersection

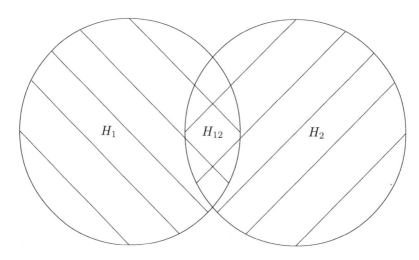

Figure 2.2   Visualization of two null hypotheses H_1 and H_2 and their intersection H_{12} using a Venn-type diagram.

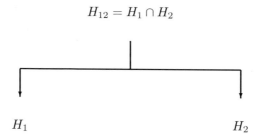

Figure 2.3   Schematic diagram of the closure principle for two null hypotheses H_1 and H_2 and their intersection.

hypotheses. In particular, different tests can be used for different hypotheses. For the final inference, an elementary null hypothesis H_i is rejected if and only if all intersection hypotheses implying H_i are rejected by their individual tests at local level α, too. It can be shown that the above procedure controls the familywise error rate strongly at level α (Marcus et al. 1976). Following the example below, a proof is sketched.

Multiple comparison procedures based on the closure principle are called *closed test procedures* below. Operationally, closed test procedures are performed as follows:

(i) Define a set $\mathcal{H} = \{H_1, \ldots, H_m\}$ of elementary hypotheses.

(ii) Construct the closure set

$$\bar{\mathcal{H}} = \left\{ H_I = \bigcap_{i \in I} H_i : I \subseteq \{1, \ldots, m\}, H_I \neq \emptyset \right\}$$

of all non-empty intersection hypotheses H_I.

(iii) For each intersection hypothesis $H_I \in \bar{\mathcal{H}}$ find a suitable (local) α-level test.

(iv) Reject H_i, if all hypotheses $H_I \in \bar{\mathcal{H}}$ with $i \in I$ are rejected, each at (local) level α.

If a closed test procedure is performed, adjusted p-values q_i for the null hypotheses H_i are computed as follows. An elementary null hypothesis H_i is only rejected, if all $H_I \in \bar{\mathcal{H}}$ with $i \in I$ are rejected, and the maximum p-value from this set needs to be less than or equal to α. Let p_I denote the p-value for a given intersection hypothesis $H_I, I \subseteq \{1, \ldots, m\}$. Then the adjusted p-value for H_i is formally defined as

$$q_i = \max_{I:i \in I} p_I, \quad i = 1, \ldots, m. \tag{2.2}$$

Example 2.1.   We provide an example of the closure principle with $m = 3$ hypotheses in Figure 2.4. Accordingly, we have three hypotheses of interest in the family $\mathcal{H} = \{H_1, H_2, H_3\}$. These three hypotheses could involve, for example, the comparison of three treatments with a control, although the following considerations are generic. This completes step 1 from above. For step 2, we need to consider all intersection hypotheses $H_I = \bigcap_{i \in I} H_i, I \subseteq \{1, \ldots, m\}$. In this example, $m = 3$ and four additional intersection hypotheses have to be considered to obtain the closed hypotheses set. Specifically, the full closure $\bar{\mathcal{H}} = \{H_1, H_2, H_3, H_{12}, H_{13}, H_{23}, H_{123}\}$ contains all seven intersection hypotheses, where $H_{ij} = H_i \cap H_j, 1 \leq i \neq j \leq 3$, and $H_{123} = H_1 \cap H_2 \cap H_3$ is the global null hypothesis. Note that $\bar{\mathcal{H}}$ is closed under intersection. That is, any intersection $H_I \cap H_{I'}$ of some $H_I, H_{I'} \in \bar{\mathcal{H}}$ is contained in $\bar{\mathcal{H}}$. For step 3, we assume suitable (local) α-level tests for each of the seven intersection hypotheses. A simple approach is to use the Bonferroni test, which is formally introduced in Section 2.3. Finally, according to step 4, we reject H_1 (while controlling the familywise error rate strongly at level α) if H_{123}, H_{12}, H_{13} and H_1 are all rejected by their α-level tests. Similarly, we reject H_2 if H_{123}, H_{12}, H_{23} and H_2 are all rejected, and we reject H_3 if H_{123}, H_{13}, H_{23} and H_3 are all rejected. In Figure 2.4, the arrows linking two hypotheses at a time reflect that the hypotheses are nested, where the smallest hypothesis H_{123} is drawn on top. For example, the arrow between H_1 and H_{12} with H_1 drawn one level below H_{12} indicates that $H_1 \supseteq H_{12}$ and H_1 can only be rejected if H_{12} is also rejected (coherence property, see Section 2.1.2).   □

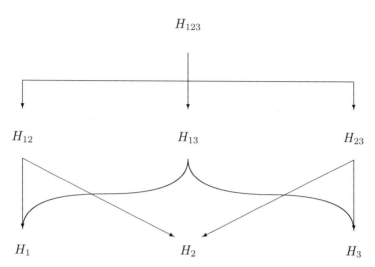

$$H_{123}$$

$$H_{12} \qquad H_{13} \qquad H_{23}$$

$$H_1 \qquad H_2 \qquad H_3$$

Figure 2.4 Schematic diagram of the closure principle for three null hypotheses $H_1, H_2,$ and H_3 and their intersections.

The closure principle can be seen to control the familywise error rate in the example above as follows. First, recall that the familywise error rate is the probability of rejecting at least one null hypothesis incorrectly. We wish to control this probability at level α, regardless of which set $M_0 \subseteq M = \{1, 2, 3\}$ of null hypotheses happens to be true. Suppose, in the example above, that H_{12} happens to be true. Then, $M_0 = \{1, 2\}$ and a Type I error occurs if either H_1 or H_2 is rejected.

If the closure principle is used, H_1 is rejected if and only if H_{123}, H_{12}, H_{13} and H_1 are all rejected. Note that the set of experiments for which $H_{123}, H_{12},$ H_{13} and H_1 are all rejected is a subset of the set of experiments for which H_{12} is rejected. Mathematically, $\{H_1$ rejected using closure$\} = \{H_{123}$ rejected$\} \cap$ $\{H_{12}$ rejected$\} \cap \{H_{13}$ rejected$\} \cap \{H_1$ rejected$\} \subseteq \{H_{12}$ rejected$\}$.

Similarly, H_2 is rejected if and only if H_{123}, H_{12}, H_{23} and H_2 are all rejected. Note that the set of experiments for which H_{123}, H_{12}, H_{23} and H_2 are all rejected is also a subset of the set of experiments for which H_{12} is rejected. Mathematically, $\{H_2$ rejected using closure$\} = \{H_{123}$ rejected$\} \cap \{H_{12}$ rejected$\} \cap$ $\{H_{23}$ rejected$\} \cap \{H_2$ rejected$\} \subseteq \{H_{12}$ rejected$\}$.

Since both

$$\{H_1 \text{ rejected using closure}\} \subseteq \{H_{12} \text{ rejected}\}$$

and

$$\{H_2 \text{ rejected using closure}\} \subseteq \{H_{12} \text{ rejected}\},$$

it follows that

$$\{\{H_1 \text{ rejected using closure}\} \cup \{H_2 \text{ rejected using closure}\}\}$$
$$\subseteq \{H_{12} \text{ rejected}\}$$

and therefore that

$$\mathbb{P}\left(\{H_1 \text{ rejected using closure}\} \cup \{H_2 \text{ rejected using closure}\}\right)$$
$$\leq \mathbb{P}\left(H_{12} \text{ rejected}\right) = \alpha.$$

Hence the method controls the familywise error rate at level less than or equal to α when the true null state of nature is H_{12}. An analogous argument shows that we have familywise error rate control when the true state of nature is H_{13}, H_{23}, or H_{123}. This argument also clarifies why all intersection hypotheses have to be tested: One needs to protect oneself against every possible combination of true and false nulls, if one wishes to control the familywise error rate in the strong sense.

The closure principle is a flexible construction method which can be tailored to a variety of applications. In particular, it provides a large degree of flexibility to map the difference in importance as well as the relationship between the various study objectives onto an adequate multiple test procedure. Many common multiple comparison procedures are in fact closed test procedures, such as the step-down procedures of Holm (1979a), Shaffer (1986), and Westfall and Young (1993), *fixed sequence tests* (Maurer, Hothorn, and Lehmacher 1995; Westfall and Krishen 2001), *fallback procedures* (Wiens 2003; Wiens and Dmitrienko 2005) and *gatekeeping procedures* (Bauer, Röhmel, Maurer, and Hothorn 1998; Westfall and Krishen 2001; Dmitrienko, Offen, and Westfall 2003). One disadvantage of the closure principle is that related simultaneous confidence intervals for the parameters of interest θ_i are difficult to derive and often have limited practical use; see Strassburger and Bretz (2008) for a recent discussion.

Note that for the closure principle the number of operations is in general of order 2^m, where m is the number of hypotheses of interest. It is often useful to find *shortcut procedures* that can reduce the number of operations to the order of m in the best case scenario (Grechanovsky and Hochberg 1999). The aim of shortcut procedures is to reach decisions for the elementary hypotheses, but not necessarily for the entire closure test. By construction, the decisions resulting from a shortcut procedure coincide with those of a closed test procedure. Shortcut procedures thus reduce the computational demand, which can be substantial for large numbers m of hypotheses and/or if resampling-based tests are used together with the closure principle. We refer to Romano and Wolf (2005), Hommel, Bretz, and Maurer (2007), Westfall and Tobias (2007), and Brannath and Bretz (2010) for further details. Related graphical approaches for sequentially rejective closed test procedures have been described by Bretz, Maurer, Brannath, and Posch (2009b); Bretz et al. (2010) and Burman, Sonesson, and Guilbaud (2009). Shortcut procedures will become essential in Chapters 3 and 4, where we use the **multcomp** package in

R, which implements efficient methods to reduce the complexity of the underlying closed test procedures. Related details are described in Sections 4.1.2 and 4.2.2, where we consider closed test procedures based on max-t tests in the form of Equation (2.1) for hypotheses satisfying the free and restricted combination condition, respectively.

2.2.4 Partitioning principle

The *partitioning principle* was formally introduced by Finner and Strassburger (2002), with early ideas dating back to Takeuchi (1973, 2010), Stefansson et al. (1988) and Hayter and Hsu (1994). Using the partitioning principle, one can derive powerful multiple test procedures and simultaneous confidence intervals, which otherwise would be difficult to obtain when applying the closure principle. The key idea of the partition principle is to partition the parameter space into disjoint subsets and test each partition element with a suitable test at level α. Because the partition elements are disjoint to each other, only one of them contains the true parameter vector and can lead to a Type I error. Hence, test procedures based on the partitioning principle strongly control the familywise error rate at level α.

To motivate the partitioning principle, we consider again the problem from Section 2.2.3 of comparing two treatments with a control. As before, let $\theta_i = \mu_i - \mu_0, i = 1, 2$, denote the parameters of interest. Let further $\Theta = \mathbb{R}^2$ denote the parameter space with $\boldsymbol{\theta} = (\theta_1, \theta_2) \in \Theta$. Recall the two hypotheses of interest, $H_i = \{\boldsymbol{\theta} \in \mathbb{R}^2 : \theta_i \leq 0\}$, $i = 1, 2$, and let $K_i = \Theta \setminus H_i$ denote the associated alternative hypotheses. Figure 2.1 visualizes the hypotheses H_1 and H_2 as subsets of the real plane (the parameter space). We now partition the parameter space Θ into the following sets, see also Figure 2.5: $\Theta_1 = H_1$, $\Theta_2 = H_2 \cap K_1$, and $\Theta_3 = K_1 \cap K_2$. Since $\Theta_i, i = 1, 2, 3$, are disjoint and $\Theta_1 \cup \Theta_2 \cup \Theta_3 = \Theta$, these sets constitute a partition of the parameter space Θ. The true parameter vector $\boldsymbol{\theta}$ thus lies in one and only one of the disjoint subsets Θ_i. Applying tests at (local) level α to each of these subsets therefore leads to a multiple test procedure which controls the familywise error rate in the strong sense at level α. Note that the resulting test procedure is at least as powerful as the corresponding closed test procedure based on H_1 and H_2, because it is sufficient to control the Type I error rate over $\Theta_1 = H_1$ and the smaller subspace $\Theta_2 \subsetneq H_2$. In addition, a confidence set for the parameter vector $\boldsymbol{\theta}$ is obtained by intersecting the complementary regions of those hypotheses, which have been rejected.

Note that the interpretation of Θ_1 is the same as of H_1 ("treatment 1 is not better than the control"). However, the interpretation of Θ_2 ("treatment 2 is not better than the control, but treatment 1 is") has changed as compared with that of H_2 ("treatment 2 is not better than the control"). There are many possibilities for partitioning the parameter space and it is not always clear which partition to apply for a given test problem. In Figure 2.5 we illustrate one example of partitioning the real plane (and which has a straightforward interpretation, as described above). Other partitions may give similar or even additional information about the parameter vector $\boldsymbol{\theta}$.

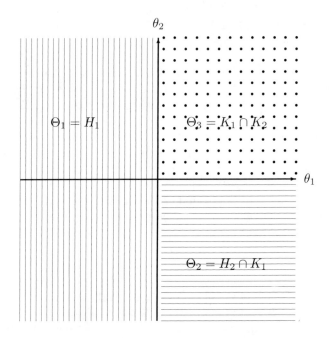

Figure 2.5 Partitioning principle for two null hypotheses H_1 and H_2.

The previous example illustrates the basic partitioning principle for two hypotheses. In the general case of m hypotheses $H_1, \ldots, H_m$, the partitioning principle can be performed operationally as follows:

(i) Choose an appropriate partition $\{\Theta_\ell : \ell \in L\}$ of the parameter space Θ for some index set L.

(ii) Test each Θ_ℓ with an α-level test.

(iii) Reject the null hypothesis H_i if all Θ_ℓ with $\Theta_\ell \cap H_i \neq \emptyset$ are rejected.

(iv) The union of all retained Θ_ℓ constitute a confidence set for $\boldsymbol{\theta}$ at level $1 - \alpha$.

For extensions of the basic partitioning principle we refer to Finner and Strassburger (2002). Applications of the partitioning principle have been investigated for a number of test problems, such as dose response analyses (Hsu and Berger 1999; Bretz, Hothorn, and Hsu 2003; Liu, Hsu, and Ruberg 2007b; Strassburger, Bretz, and Finner 2007), multiple outcome analyses (Liu and Hsu 2009), intersection union tests (Strassburger et al. 2004), equivalence tests (Finner, Giani, and Strassburger 2006), and simultaneous confidence intervals for step-up and step-down procedures (Finner and Strassburger 2006; Strassburger and Bretz 2008).

2.3 Methods based on Bonferroni's inequality

The Bonferroni method is probably the best known multiplicity adjustment. Although more powerful multiple comparison procedures exist, the Bonferroni test continues to be very popular because of its simplicity and its mild assumptions. In this section we describe the Bonferroni test, a stepwise extension (Holm 1979a) and discuss further topics related to these methods. We also describe briefly some software implementations in R, leaving the details for Section 3.3.

2.3.1 Bonferroni test

The *Bonferroni test* is a single-step procedure, which compares the unadjusted p-values $p_1, \ldots, p_m$ with the common threshold α/m, where m is the number of hypotheses under investigation. Equivalently, a null hypothesis $H_i, i \in M$, is rejected, if the adjusted p-value $q_i = \min\{mp_i, 1\} \leq \alpha$. Here, the minimum is used to ensure that the resulting adjusted p-value q_i is not larger than 1. The strong control of the familywise error rate follows directly from Bonferroni's inequality

$$\mathbb{P}(V > 0) = \mathbb{P}\left(\bigcup_{i \in M_0} \{q_i \leq \alpha\} \right) \leq \sum_{i \in M_0} \mathbb{P}(q_i \leq \alpha) \leq m_0 \alpha/m \leq \alpha, \qquad (2.3)$$

where the probability expressions are conditional on $\bigcap_{i \in M_0} H_i$ and $M_0 \subseteq M$ denotes the set of $m_0 = |M_0|$ true null hypotheses (recall Table 2.1 for the related notation).

Example 2.2. Consider the following numerical example with $m = 3$ null hypotheses being tested at level $\alpha = 0.025$. Let $p_1 = 0.01, p_2 = 0.015$, and $p_3 = 0.005$ denote the unadjusted p-values. Because $p_3 < \alpha/3 = 0.0083$, but $p_1, p_2 > \alpha/3$, only the null hypothesis H_3 is rejected. Alternatively, the adjusted p-values $q_1 = 0.03, q_2 = 0.045$, and $q_3 = 0.015$ can be compared with $\alpha = 0.025$, leading to the same test decisions. □

A convenient way to perform the Bonferroni test in R is to call the `p.adjust` function from the **stats** package. Its use is self-explanantory. To calculate the adjusted p-values q_i in the previous example, we first define a vector containing the unadjusted p-values and subsequently call the `p.adjust` function as follows:

```
R> p <- c(0.01, 0.015, 0.005)
R> p.adjust(p, "bonferroni")
```

```
[1] 0.030 0.045 0.015
```

In Section 3.3 we provide a detailed description of the **multcomp** package in

R, which provides an interface to the multiplicity adjustments implemented in the `p.adjust` function and also allows one to perform more sophisticated multiple comparison procedures.

The Bonferroni method is a very general approach, which is valid for any correlation structure among the test statistics. However, the Bonferroni test is conservative in the sense that other test procedures exist, which reject at least as many hypotheses as the Bonferroni test (often at the cost of additional assumptions on the joint distribution of the test statistics). In the following we describe some improvements or generalizations of the Bonferroni approach.

2.3.2 Holm procedure

Holm (1979a) introduced a multiple comparison procedure, which uniformly improves the Bonferroni approach. The *Holm procedure* is a step-down procedure, which basically consists of repeatedly applying Bonferroni's inequality while testing the hypotheses in a data-dependent order. Let $p_{(1)} \leq \ldots \leq p_{(m)}$ denote the ordered unadjusted p-values with associated hypotheses $H_{(1)}, \ldots, H_{(m)}$. Then, $H_{(i)}$ is rejected if $p_{(j)} \leq \alpha/(m - j + 1), j = 1, \ldots, i$. That is, $H_{(i)}$ is rejected if $p_{(i)} \leq \alpha/(m - i + 1)$ and all hypotheses $H_{(j)}$ preceding $H_{(i)}$ are also rejected. Adjusted p-values for the Holm procedure are given by

$$q_{(i)} = \min\{1, \max[(m - i + 1)p_{(i)}, q_{(i-1)}]\}. \tag{2.4}$$

Alternatively, the Holm procedure can be described by the following sequentially rejective test procedure. Start testing the null hypothesis $H_{(1)}$ associated with the smallest p-value $p_{(1)}$. If $p_{(1)} > \alpha/m$, the procedure stops and no hypothesis is rejected. Otherwise, $H_{(1)}$ is rejected and the procedure continues testing $H_{(2)}$ at the larger significance level $\alpha/(m-1)$. These steps are repeated until either the first non-rejection occurs or all null hypotheses $H_{(1)}, \ldots, H_{(m)}$ are rejected.

Example 2.3.   Consider again the p-values from Example 2.2. Since $p_{(1)} = 0.005 < 0.0083 = \alpha/3$, $H_{(1)} = H_3$ is rejected at $\alpha = 0.025$. At the second step, $p_{(2)} = 0.01 < 0.0125 = \alpha/2$ and $H_{(2)} = H_1$ is also rejected. At the final step, $p_{(3)} = 0.015 < 0.025 = \alpha$ and $H_{(3)} = H_2$ is also rejected. Alternatively, the adjusted p-values are calculated as $q_{(1)} = 0.015, q_{(2)} = 0.02$, and $q_{(3)} = 0.02$, which are all smaller than $\alpha = 0.025$ and thus lead to the same test decisions. Using the `p.adjust` function introduced in Section 2.3.1, we obtain these adjusted p-values by calling

```
R> p.adjust(p, "holm")
```

```
[1] 0.020 0.020 0.015
```

Note that $q_{(3)} = 0.02$ (and not 0.015, as one might expect) due to the monotonicity enforcement induced by the maximum argument in (2.4).   □

It becomes clear from this example that the Holm procedure is a step-down procedure, which by construction rejects all hypotheses rejected by the Bonferroni test and possibly others. We now give a different perspective on the Holm procedure by considering the closure principle from Section 2.2.3. For null hypotheses $H_1, \ldots, H_m$ satisfying the free combination condition (Section 2.1.2), the Holm procedure is a shortcut of the closure principle when applying the Bonferroni test to each intersection hypothesis $H_I = \bigcap_{i \in I} H_i, I \subseteq \{1, \ldots, m\}$ (Holm 1979a). That is, the Holm procedure leads to the same decisions for the elementary hypotheses $H_1, \ldots, H_m$ as a Bonferroni-based closed test procedure. To see this, consider again the example from Section 2.2.3 comparing two treatments with a control. The related closure principle for the two null hypotheses H_1 and H_2 is shown in Figure 2.3. Assume now that the Bonferroni method is used to test the intersection hypothesis $H_{12} = H_1 \cap H_2$, that is, H_{12} is rejected if $\min(p_1, p_2) \leq \alpha/2$. If H_{12} is rejected, then one of the elementary hypotheses H_1 and H_2 is immediately rejected as well and only the remaining hypothesis needs to be tested at level α: If, say, $p_1 < \alpha/2$, then trivially $p_1 < \alpha$ and H_1 is rejected; H_2 remains to be tested at level α. More generally, if $H_I = \bigcap_{i \in I} H_i, I \subseteq M$, is rejected, then there exists an index $i^* \in I$ such that $p_{i^*} \leq \alpha/|I|$ and all hypotheses H_J with $i^* \in J \subseteq I$ are also rejected, because $|J| \leq |I|$ and consequently $p_{i^*} \leq \alpha/|I| \leq \alpha/|J|$.

Because the Holm procedure is based on the conservative Bonferroni inequality (2.3), more powerful step-down procedures can be obtained by accounting for the stochastic dependencies between the test statistics. In Section 4.1.2 we discuss a parametric extension of the Holm procedure based on max-t tests in the form (2.1). We also show how to implement these methods using R.

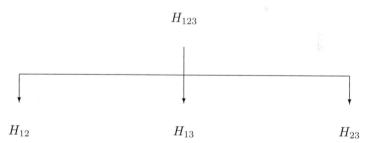

H_{123}

H_{12} H_{13} H_{23}

Figure 2.6   Schematic diagram of the closure principle for the three null hypotheses $H_{ij} \colon \mu_i = \mu_j, 1 \leq i < j \leq 3$.

If the null hypotheses $H_1, \ldots, H_m$ satisfy the restricted combination condition, however, the Holm procedure is still applicable, but conservative. To see this, consider all pairwise comparisons of three treatments means μ_1, μ_2, and μ_3, resulting in $m = 3$ null hypotheses $H_{ij} \colon \mu_i = \mu_j$. The related closure principle for the three null hypotheses H_{12}, H_{13}, and H_{23} is shown in Figure 2.6, where $H_{123} \colon \mu_1 = \mu_2 = \mu_3$ is the only non-trivial intersection hypothesis. Applying the Bonferroni test leads to the rejection of H_{123} if $\min(p_1, p_2, p_3) < \alpha/3$. Once H_{123} has been rejected, one of the elementary hypotheses is immediately rejected as well and only the two remaining hypotheses need to be tested at level α. Note that for the ordered set of p-values $(p_{(1)}, p_{(2)}, p_{(3)})$ the Holm procedure would apply the significance thresholds $(\alpha/3, \alpha/2, \alpha)$, whereas the thresholds $(\alpha/3, \alpha, \alpha)$ would suffice, as seen from this example. Note also that in some cases the Holm procedure may not be coherent under the restricted combination condition (Hommel and Bretz 2008).

Shaffer (1986) extended the Holm procedure, utilizing logical restrictions to improve the power of closed tests. Her method is a "truncated" closed test procedure: Closed testing is performed, in sequence $H_{(1)}, H_{(2)}, \ldots$ corresponding to the ordered p-values, and testing stops at the first insignificance. Truncation ensures that $H_{(i')}$ cannot be rejected if $H_{(i)}$ is not rejected, for $i' > i$. Without truncation, a closed test procedure can result in the possibly undesirable outcome that $H_{(i')}$ is rejected and $H_{(i)}$ is not rejected, for $i' > i$; see Bergmann and Hommel (1988), Hommel and Bernhard (1999), and Westfall and Tobias (2007) for details. When the tests satisfy the free combinations condition, all these procedures reduce to the ordinary Holm procedure.

Although based on the conservative Bonferroni inequality, Shaffer's method can be much more powerful than standard methods when combinations are restricted. In Section 4.2.2, we discuss a parametric extension of Shaffer's method (called the extended Shaffer-Royen procedure by Westfall and Tobias (2007)) that is yet more powerful than Shaffer's method. The increase in power comes from using specific dependence information rather than the conservative Bonferroni inequality. We also show how to implement this powerful method using the **multcomp** package in R.

2.3.3 Further topics

In this section we describe additional extensions of the procedures by Bonferroni and Holm. Simultaneous confidence intervals compatible with the Bonferroni test are easily obtained by computing the marginal confidence intervals at the adjusted significance levels α/m. For the Holm procedure, such confidence intervals are more difficult to construct (Section 2.1.2). We refer to Strassburger and Bretz (2008) and Guilbaud (2008), who independently applied the partitioning principle from Section 2.2.4 to derive compatible simultaneous confidence intervals for the Holm procedure and other Bonferroni-based closed test procedures.

If the test statistics were independent, the familywise error rate would become

$$\text{FWER} = \mathbb{P}(V > 0) = 1 - \mathbb{P}(V = 0) = 1 - (1 - \alpha)^m.$$

This gives the motivation for the Šidák (1967) approach, which rejects a null hypothesis H_i, if $p_i \leq 1 - (1 - \alpha)^{1/m}$, or, equivalently, if the adjusted p-value $q_i = 1 - (1 - p_i)^m \leq \alpha$. The Šidák approach also holds for non-negatively correlated test statistics (Tong 1980). Note that the Šidák approach is more powerful than the Bonferroni test, although the gain in power is marginal in practice. A further modification of the Bonferroni method, which has attracted substantial research interest, is based on the Simes inequality described in Section 2.4. Further improvements of the Bonferroni method, which incorporate stochastic dependencies in the data, are parametric approaches described in Chapter 3 and resampling-based approaches reviewed in Section 5.1.

It follows from the inequality (2.3) that the Bonferroni test controls the familywise error rate strongly at level α or less, that is, FWER $\leq m_0 \alpha / m \leq \alpha$. If the number m_0 of true null hypotheses was known, more powerful procedures could be obtained by applying the Bonferroni test at level $m_0 \alpha / m$ instead of α. Several methods are available to estimate m_0 and five of them were compared in Hsueh, Chen, and Kodell (2003). The authors concluded that the approach proposed by Benjamini and Hochberg (2000) gives satisfactory empirical results. The latter considered the slopes of the lines passing the points $(m + 1, 1)$ and $(i, p_{(i)})$, and took the lowest slope estimator to approximate m_0. More recently, Finner and Gontscharuk (2009) derived conditions which ensure familywise error rate control of Bonferroni-based test procedures using plug-in estimates similar to those proposed by Schweder and Spjøtvoll (1982) and Storey (2002).

Westfall, Kropf, and Finos (2004) described weighted methods that are useful when some hypotheses H_i are deemed more important than others. For example, in clinical trials the various patient outcomes might be ranked a priori, and the test procedure designed to give more power to the more important hypotheses. The simplest weighted multiple comparison procedure is the weighted Bonferroni test, discussed in, for example, Rosenthal and Rubin (1983). The weighted Bonferroni test divides the overall significance level α into portions $w_1\alpha, \ldots, w_m\alpha$, such that $\sum_i w_i \alpha = \alpha$. Accordingly, an elementary hypothesis H_i is rejected if $p_i \leq w_1\alpha$. Holm (1979a) introduced the following weighted test procedure, which extends the weighted Bonferroni test described above. Order the weighted p-values $\tilde{p}_i = p_i / w_i$ as $\tilde{p}_{(1)} \leq \ldots \leq \tilde{p}_{(m)}$, where $\tilde{p}_{(j)} = \tilde{p}_{i_j}$ (that is, i_j denotes the index of the j-th ordered weighted p-value). Define the sets $S_j = \{i_j, \ldots, i_m\}$, $j = 1, \ldots, m$. Let $H^w_{(j)}$ denote the hypothesis corresponding to $\tilde{p}_{(j)}$. The weighted Holm procedure rejects $H^w_{(j)}$, if $\tilde{p}_{(i)} \leq \alpha / \sum_{h \in S_i} w_h$, for all $i = 1, \ldots, j$. This method controls the familywise error rate strongly at level α, and when the weights are equal, it reduces to the ordinary Holm procedure. Closed test procedures based on weighted Bonferroni tests have recently attracted much attention for the analysis of multiple outcome variables; see Dmitrienko et al. (2003), Hommel et al. (2007), and Bretz et al. (2009b).

2.4 Methods based on Simes' inequality

Simes (1986) proposed the following modification of the Bonferroni method to test the global intersection hypothesis $H = \bigcap_{i \in M} H_i$. Let again $p_{(1)} \leq \ldots \leq p_{(m)}$ denote the ordered unadjusted p-values with associated hypotheses

$H_{(1)}, \ldots, H_{(m)}$. Using the Simes test, one rejects H if there is an index $j \in M = \{1, \ldots, m\}$, such that $p_{(j)} \leq j\alpha/m$. However, one cannot assess the elementary hypotheses H_i with the Simes test. In particular, one cannot reject $H_{(i)}$ if $p_{(i)} \leq i\alpha/m$ for some $i \in M$, because the familywise error rate is not controlled in this case (Hommel 1988).

By construction, the Simes test is more powerful than the Bonferroni test in the sense that whenever H is rejected by the latter it will also be rejected by the former, but not vice versa. Figure 2.7 compares the rejection regions of the Bonferroni and the Simes tests for $m = 2$. Recall that when $m = 2$ the Bonferroni test rejects the global intersection hypothesis H if either $p_1 \leq \alpha/2$ or $p_2 \leq \alpha/2$. The Simes test rejects H if either $p_{(1)} \leq \alpha/2$ or $p_{(2)} \leq \alpha$. As seen from Figure 2.7, the Simes test "adds" the square $[\alpha/2, \alpha] \times [\alpha/2, \alpha]$ to the rejection region of the Bonferroni test and is therefore more powerful.

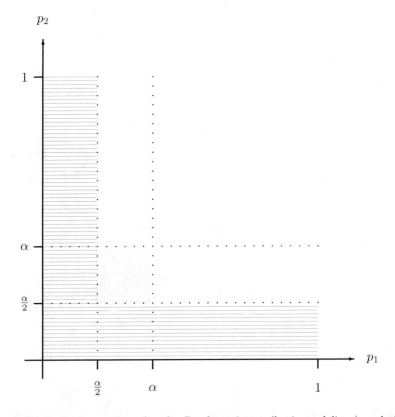

Figure 2.7   Rejection regions for the Bonferroni test (horizontal lines) and the Simes test (horizontal and vertical lines).

To illustrate the impact on the (disjunctive) power, Figure 2.8 displays 100 simulated pairs of independent p-values (p_1, p_2) under a given alternative. Setting $\alpha = 0.1$, the Bonferroni test rejects in those 88 cases, where in Figure 2.8 the dots lie in the lower left "L-shaped" region $\{p_1 \le \alpha/2\} \cup \{p_2 \le \alpha/2\}$. The Simes test rejects in one additional case, where $(p_1, p_2) = (0.0807, 0.0602)$, confirming its slight power advantage. In the remaining 11 cases neither the Bonferroni nor the Simes test rejects.

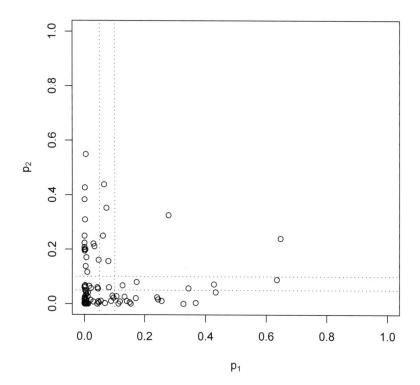

Figure 2.8 Illustration of the power difference for the Bonferroni and Simes tests by plotting 100 pairs of independent p-values (p_1, p_2).

Note that the power advantage of the Simes test comes at the cost of additional assumptions on the underlying dependency structure. Simes (1986) proved that for his test FWER $= \alpha$ under independence of $p_1, \ldots, p_m$. If the independence assumption is not met, the Type I error rate control is not always clear. In many practically relevant cases the inflation in size is marginal (Samuel-Cahn 1996), although pathological counter-examples exist, where the impact can be substantial (Hommel 1983). For one-sided tests, it can be shown that the Simes test controls the familywise error rate if, for example, the test statistics are multivariate normally distributed with non-negative correlations or multivariate t distributed with the associated normals having non-negative correlations, as long as $\alpha < 1/2$. We refer to Sarkar and Chang (1997) and Sarkar (1998) for further results.

Hochberg (1988) proposed a step-up extension of the Simes test, which allows one to make inferences about the elementary null hypotheses $H_i, i \in M$. The Hochberg procedure can be seen as a reversed Holm procedure, since it uses the same critical values, but in a reversed test sequence: $H_{(i)}$ is rejected if there is a $j = i, \ldots, m$, such that $p_{(j)} \leq \alpha/(m - j + 1)$. Adjusted p-values for the Hochberg procedure are given by

$$q_{(i)} = \min\{1, \min[(m - i + 1)p_{(i)}, q_{(i+1)}]\}.$$

Alternatively, the Hochberg procedure can be described by the following sequentially rejective test procedure. Start testing the null hypothesis $H_{(m)}$ associated with the largest p-value $p_{(m)}$. If $p_{(m)} \leq \alpha$, the procedure stops and all hypothesis $H_{(1)}, \ldots, H_{(m)}$ are rejected. Otherwise, $H_{(m)}$ is retained and the procedure continues testing $H_{(m-1)}$ at the smaller significance level $\alpha/2$. If $p_{(m-1)} \leq \alpha/2$, the procedure stops and all hypothesis $H_{(1)}, \ldots, H_{(m-1)}$ are rejected. These steps are repeated until either the first rejection occurs or all null hypotheses $H_{(1)}, \ldots, H_{(m)}$ are retained. By construction, the Hochberg procedure is more powerful than the Holm procedure.

Example 2.4.   Consider the following numerical example with $m = 4$ null hypotheses tested at the significance level $\alpha = 0.05$. Let $p_1 = 0.022, p_2 = 0.02$, $p_3 = 0.01$, and $p_4 = 0.09$ be the unadjusted p-values. Consider first the Holm procedure. Since $p_{(1)} = p_3 = 0.01 < 0.0125 = \alpha/4$, $H_{(1)} = H_3$ is rejected. At the second step, $p_{(2)} = p_2 = 0.02 > 0.0167 = \alpha/3$ and the Holm procedure stops with no further rejections. The Hochberg procedure, however, starts with the largest p-value, steps through the ordered p-values, and stops with the first significant result. Because $p_{(4)} = p_4 = 0.09 > 0.05 = \alpha$ but $p_{(3)} = p_1 = 0.022 < 0.025 = \alpha/2$, the Hochberg procedure rejects H_1, H_2, and H_3 but not $H_{(4)} = H_4$. Table 2.2 summarizes this example and gives the associated adjusted p-values.   □

Hommel (1988) introduced an improved procedure by applying the Simes test to each intersection hypothesis of a closed test procedure. This procedure can be shown to be uniformly more powerful than the Hochberg procedure (Hommel 1989). As an example consider the case $m = 3$ and assume that $p_1 \leq p_2 \leq p_3$. The Hochberg procedure then rejects H_1 if any of the events

$$\{p_3 \leq \alpha\}$$
$$\text{or} \quad \{p_2 \leq \alpha/2 \text{ and } p_1 \leq \alpha/2\}$$
$$\text{or} \quad \{p_1 \leq \alpha/3\}$$

		Threshold	Decision		Adjusted p-value	
i	$p_{(i)}$	$\alpha/(4-i+1)$	Holm	Hochberg	Holm	Hochberg
1	0.01	0.0125	Rej.	Rej.	0.04	0.04
2	0.02	0.0167	N.R.	Rej.	0.06	0.044
3	0.022	0.025	N.R.	Rej.	0.06	0.044
4	0.09	0.05	N.R.	N.R.	0.09	0.09

Table 2.2 Comparison of the Holm and Hochberg procedures for $m = 4$ hypotheses and $\alpha = 0.05$. Rej. = rejection, N.R. = no rejection.

is true. In contrast, the procedure by Hommel rejects H_1 if any of the events

$$\{p_3 \le \alpha\}$$
$$\text{or} \quad \{p_2 \le 2\alpha/3 \text{ and } p_1 \le \alpha/2\}$$
$$\text{or} \quad \{p_1 \le \alpha/3\}$$

is true. Thus, if $\alpha/2 < p_2 \le 2\alpha/3$ and $p_1 \le \alpha/2$, the Hommel procedure rejects H_1, but the Hochberg procedure does not.

Both the Hochberg and the Hommel procedure are available in R with the p.adjust function introduced in Section 2.3.1. For example, calling

```
R> p <- c(0.01, 0.02, 0.022, 0.09)
R> p.adjust(p, "hochberg")
```

```
[1] 0.040 0.044 0.044 0.090
```

gives the adjusted p-values from Table 2.2. Similarly, the Hommel procedure is available with

```
R> p.adjust(p, "hommel")
```

```
[1] 0.030 0.040 0.044 0.090
```

Note that in this example the Hommel procedure leads to smaller adjusted p-values for H_1 and H_2 than the Hochberg procedure, reflecting the previous comment about its power advantage.

CHAPTER 3

Multiple Comparison Procedures in Parametric Models

In this chapter we introduce a general framework for multiple hypotheses testing in parametric and semi-parametric models. This chapter provides the theoretical basis for the applications analyzed in Chapter 4. In Section 3.1 we review briefly the standard linear model theory and show how to perform multiple comparisons in this framework, including analysis-of-variance (ANOVA), analysis-of-covariance (ANCOVA) and regression models as special cases. We extend the basic approaches from Chapter 2 by using inherent distributional assumptions, particularly by accounting for the structural correlation between the test statistics, thus achieving larger power. In addition, we revisit the linear regression example from Chapter 1 to illustrate the resulting methods. In Section 3.2 we extend the previous linear model framework and introduce multiple comparison procedures for general parametric models relying on standard asymptotic normality results. The methods apply, for example, to generalized linear models, linear and non-linear mixed-effects models as well as survival data. Again, the use of the inherent stochastic dependencies leads to powerful methods. The **multcomp** package in R provides a convenient interface to perform multiple comparisons for the parametric models considered in Sections 3.1 and 3.2. An in-depth introduction to the **multcomp** package is given in Section 3.3. Detailed examples to illustrate and extend the results from this chapter are left for Chapter 4.

3.1 General linear models

In Section 3.1.1 we introduce the canonical framework for multiple hypotheses testing in general linear models. We refer to several standard results from the theory of linear models which will be used subsequently; see Searle (1971) for a detailed mathematical treatise of this subject. In Section 3.1.2 we revisit the linear regression example from Chapter 1 to illustrate some of the results using R.

3.1.1 Multiple comparisons in linear models

Multiple comparisons in linear models have been considered previously in the literature; see, for example, the standard textbooks from Hochberg and Tamhane (1987) and Hsu (1996). Here, we follow the description from Bretz,

Hothorn, and Westfall (2008a) and consider the common general linear model

$$\mathbf{y} = \mathbf{X}\boldsymbol{\beta} + \boldsymbol{\varepsilon}, \tag{3.1}$$

where $\mathbf{y} = (y_1, \ldots, y_n)^\top$ denotes the $n \times 1$ vector of observations, $\mathbf{X} = (x_{ij})_{ij}$ denotes the fixed and known $n \times p$ design matrix, and $\boldsymbol{\beta} = (\beta_1, \ldots, \beta_p)^\top$ denotes the fixed and unknown parameter vector. The random, unobservable $n \times 1$ error vector $\boldsymbol{\varepsilon}$ is assumed to follow an n-dimensional normal distribution with mean vector $\mathbf{0} = (0, \ldots, 0)^\top$ and covariance matrix $\sigma^2 \mathbf{I}_n$, $\boldsymbol{\varepsilon} \sim N_n(\mathbf{0}, \sigma^2 \mathbf{I}_n)$ for short, where N_n denotes an n-dimensional normal distribution, σ^2 the common variance, and $\mathbf{I}_n$ the identity matrix of dimension n. Model (3.1) implies that each individual observation y_i follows the linear model

$$y_i = \beta_1 x_{i1} + \ldots + \beta_p x_{ip} + \varepsilon,$$

where $\varepsilon \sim N(0, \sigma^2)$. Extensions of this linear model will be considered in Section 3.2 and a variety of applications will be discussed in Chapter 4.

Assume that we want to perform pre-specified comparisons among the parameters $\beta_1, \ldots, \beta_p$. To accomplish this, define a $p \times 1$ vector $\mathbf{c} = (c_1, \ldots, c_p)^\top$ of known constants. If the vector $\mathbf{c}$ is chosen such that $\mathbf{c}^\top \mathbf{1} = 0$, where $\mathbf{1} = (1, \ldots, 1)^\top$, it is denoted as contrast vector. The vector $\mathbf{c}$ thus reflects a single experimental comparison of interest through the linear combination $\mathbf{c}^\top \boldsymbol{\beta}$ with associated null hypothesis

$$H : \mathbf{c}^\top \boldsymbol{\beta} = a \tag{3.2}$$

for a fixed and known constant a. In the following, we refer to $\mathbf{c}^\top \boldsymbol{\beta}$ as the (linear) function of interest; all such functions are assumed to be estimable as defined below. If we have multiple experimental questions, m say, we obtain m vectors $\mathbf{c}_1, \ldots, \mathbf{c}_m$, which can be summarized by the matrix $\mathbf{C} = (\mathbf{c}_1, \ldots, \mathbf{c}_m)$, resulting in the m elementary null hypotheses

$$H_j : \mathbf{c}_j^\top \boldsymbol{\beta} = a_j, \quad j = 1, \ldots, m.$$

Example 3.1. Recall the linear regression example from Chapter 1. There we considered the multiple test problem of whether intercept or slope from a linear regression model differ significantly from zero. Based on the `thuesen` data, we want to predict the ventricular shortening velocity y from blood glucose x using the model

$$y_i = \beta_1 + \beta_2 x_i + \varepsilon_i$$

for the i-th patient, where β_1 denotes the intercept and β_2 denotes the slope. We can thus assume that the $n = 23$ individual measurements follow the linear model (3.1), where

$$
\mathbf{y} = \begin{pmatrix} 1.76 \\ 1.34 \\ 1.27 \\ \vdots \\ 1.03 \\ 1.12 \\ 1.70 \end{pmatrix}, \quad \mathbf{X} = \begin{pmatrix} 1 & 15.3 \\ 1 & 10.8 \\ 1 & 8.1 \\ \vdots & \vdots \\ 1 & 4.9 \\ 1 & 8.8 \\ 1 & 9.5 \end{pmatrix}, \quad \text{and} \quad \boldsymbol{\beta} = \begin{pmatrix} \beta_1 \\ \beta_2 \end{pmatrix}.
$$

For the **thuesen** data example we are interested in testing the $m = 2$ elementary null hypotheses

$$
H_1: \beta_1 = 0 \quad \text{and} \quad H_2: \beta_2 = 0,
$$

where

$$
\mathbf{a} = \begin{pmatrix} a_1 \\ a_2 \end{pmatrix} = \begin{pmatrix} 0 \\ 0 \end{pmatrix} \quad \text{and} \quad \mathbf{C} = \begin{pmatrix} 1 & 0 \\ 0 & 1 \end{pmatrix}
$$

in the notation from Equation (3.2).   □

Standard linear model theory provides the usual least squares estimates

$$
\hat{\boldsymbol{\beta}} = (\mathbf{X}^\top \mathbf{X})^- \mathbf{X}^\top \mathbf{y} \tag{3.3}
$$

and

$$
\hat{\sigma}^2 = \frac{(\mathbf{y} - \mathbf{X}\hat{\boldsymbol{\beta}})^\top (\mathbf{y} - \mathbf{X}\hat{\boldsymbol{\beta}})}{\nu}, \tag{3.4}
$$

where $\nu = n - \operatorname{rank}(\mathbf{X})$ and $(\mathbf{X}^\top \mathbf{X})^-$ denotes some generalized inverse of $\mathbf{X}^\top \mathbf{X}$. Under the model assumptions (3.1), $\hat{\sigma}^2$ is an unbiased estimate of σ^2. If $\operatorname{rank}(\mathbf{X}) = p$, the estimate $\hat{\boldsymbol{\beta}} = (\mathbf{X}^\top \mathbf{X})^{-1} \mathbf{X}^\top \mathbf{y}$ is also unbiased.

We can test the hypotheses H_j using the quantities

$$
t_j = \frac{\mathbf{c}_j^\top \hat{\boldsymbol{\beta}} - a_j}{\hat{\sigma} \sqrt{\mathbf{c}_j^\top (\mathbf{X}^\top \mathbf{X})^- \mathbf{c}_j}}, \quad j = 1, \ldots, m, \tag{3.5}
$$

one for each experimental question defined through $\mathbf{c}_j$. By construction, each test statistic $t_j, j = 1, \ldots, m$, follows under the null hypothesis (3.2) a central univariate t distribution with ν degrees of freedom. When the null hypothesis $H_j: \mathbf{c}_j^\top \boldsymbol{\beta} = a$ is not true, t_j follows a non-central univariate t distribution with ν degrees of freedom and noncentrality parameter

$$
\tau_j = \frac{\mathbf{c}_j^\top \boldsymbol{\beta} - a_j}{\sigma \sqrt{\mathbf{c}_j^\top (\mathbf{X}^\top \mathbf{X})^- \mathbf{c}_j}}, \quad j = 1, \ldots, m.
$$

The joint distribution of $t_1, \ldots, t_m$ is multivariate t with ν degrees of freedom and correlation matrix

$$
\mathbf{R} = \mathbf{D}\mathbf{C}^\top (\mathbf{X}^\top \mathbf{X})^- \mathbf{C}\mathbf{D},
$$

where $\mathbf{D} = \operatorname{diag}(\mathbf{c}_j^\top (\mathbf{X}^\top \mathbf{X})^- \mathbf{c}_j)^{-1/2}$. If σ is known or in the asymptotic case $\nu \to \infty$, the (limiting) multivariate normal distribution holds.

Let $u_{1-\alpha}$ denote the critical value derived from the multivariate normal or t distribution for a pre-specified significance level α. We then reject the null hypothesis H_j if $|t_j| \geq u_{1-\alpha}$. Alternatively, if q_j denotes the adjusted p-value for H_j computed from either the multivariate normal or t distribution, we reject H_j if $q_j \leq \alpha$ (recall Section 2.1.2 for a generic definition of adjusted p-values). Confidence intervals for $\mathbf{c}_j^\top \boldsymbol{\beta} - a_j$, $j = 1, \ldots, m$, with simultaneous coverage probability $1 - \alpha$ are given through

$$\left[\mathbf{c}_j^\top \hat{\boldsymbol{\beta}} - a_j - u_{1-\alpha} \hat{\sigma} \sqrt{\mathbf{c}_j^\top (\mathbf{X}^\top \mathbf{X})^- \mathbf{c}_j}; \; \mathbf{c}_j^\top \hat{\boldsymbol{\beta}} - a_j + u_{1-\alpha} \hat{\sigma} \sqrt{\mathbf{c}_j^\top (\mathbf{X}^\top \mathbf{X})^- \mathbf{c}_j} \right].$$

We obtain similar results for one-sided test problems by reformulating the null hypotheses, taking the test statistics t_j instead of their absolute values $|t_j|$, and computing the associated one-sided critical values and/or adjusted p-values. Genz and Bretz (1999, 2002, 2009) described numerical integration methods to calculate multivariate normal and t probabilities. For a general overview of these distributions we refer the reader to the books of Tong (1990); Kotz, Balakrishnan, and Johnson (2000) and Kotz and Nadarajah (2004).

The methods discussed in this section lead to powerful multiple comparison procedures. These procedures extend the classical Bonferroni method from Section 2.3.1 by considering the joint multivariate normal or t distribution of the individual test statistics (3.5). However, the methods presented here belong to the class of single-step procedures. As explained in Section 2.2.3, more powerful closed test procedures based on max-t tests of the form (2.1) can be constructed, which utilize the correlation structure involved in the joint distribution of the test statistics (either multivariate t or multivariate normal). It is the combination of the methods from this section with the closure principle described earlier, that results in powerful stepwise procedures and forms the core methodology for the application analyses in Chapter 4.

Example 3.2.   Revisiting the `thuesen` data from Example 3.1, we have $\hat{\boldsymbol{\beta}} = (1.098, 0.022)^\top$ and $\hat{\sigma} = 0.217$. In Section 3.1.2 we will extract this information from the fitted linear model in R. These numbers can also be computed using Equations (3.3) and (3.4). Plugging the estimates $\hat{\boldsymbol{\beta}}$ and $\hat{\sigma}$ into Equation (3.5) results in the test statistics $t_1 = 9.345$ and $t_2 = 2.101$ with $\nu = 21$ degrees of freedom. Based on the correlation of -0.923 between the two test statistics, we can then compute the required bivariate t probabilities for the multiplicity adjusted p-values, as shown in Section 3.1.2.   □

We conclude this section by reviewing the estimability conditions for linear functions in general linear models. We again refer to Searle (1971) for further details. A function $\mathbf{c}^\top \boldsymbol{\beta}$ is called estimable if there exists a $n \times 1$ vector $\mathbf{z}$ such that $\mathbb{E}(\mathbf{z}^\top \mathbf{y}) = \mathbb{E}(\sum_{i=1}^n z_i Y_i) = \mathbf{c}^\top \boldsymbol{\beta}$. If such a vector $\mathbf{z}$ cannot be found, the function $\mathbf{c}^\top \boldsymbol{\beta}$ is not estimable. A necessary and sufficient condition for the estimability of $\mathbf{c}^\top \boldsymbol{\beta}$ is given by

$$\mathbf{c}^\top (\mathbf{X}^\top \mathbf{X})^- \mathbf{X}^\top \mathbf{X} = \mathbf{c}^\top.$$

Further, if $\mathbf{c}^\top\boldsymbol{\beta}$ is estimable, then $\mathbb{E}\left(\mathbf{z}^\top\mathbf{y}\right) = \mathbf{c}^\top\boldsymbol{\beta}$, where

$$\mathbf{z}^\top = \mathbf{c}^\top\left(\mathbf{X}^\top\mathbf{X}\right)^-\mathbf{X}^\top.$$

Moreover, if $\mathbf{c}^\top\boldsymbol{\beta}$ is estimable, then $\mathbf{c}^\top\hat{\boldsymbol{\beta}} = \mathbf{z}^\top\mathbf{y}$ is the best linear unbiased estimator of $\mathbf{c}^\top\boldsymbol{\beta}$ and its variance

$$\mathbb{V}(\mathbf{z}^\top\mathbf{y}) = \sigma^2\mathbf{c}^\top\left(\mathbf{X}^\top\mathbf{X}\right)^-\mathbf{c}$$

does not depend on the particular choice of the generalized inverse. Thus, once the estimability of $\mathbf{c}^\top\boldsymbol{\beta}$ is confirmed, we obtain a good and unique estimate of the function $\mathbf{c}^\top\boldsymbol{\beta}$ of interest through $\mathbf{c}^\top\left(\mathbf{X}^\top\mathbf{X}\right)^-\mathbf{X}^\top\mathbf{y}$. Note that we have used this result already in Equations (3.3) and (3.5).

3.1.2 The linear regression example revisited using R

As a direct consequence of the linear model theory reviewed in Section 3.1.1, the implementation of any advanced multiple comparison procedure requires careful consideration of several individual steps. Flexible interfaces, such as the **multcomp** package in R, facilitate the use of such advanced methods. In this section we revisit the linear regression example based on the thuesen data from Chapter 1 to illustrate the key steps when using the **multcomp** package. A detailed introduction to the package is given in Section 3.3.

If the **multcomp** package was not available, we would need to make the necessary calculations step by step based on the methods from Section 3.1.1. The necessary estimates of the regression coefficients β and their covariance matrix can be extracted from the previously fitted model (see Chapter 1 for the associated lm fit) by calling

```
R> betahat <- coef(thuesen.lm)
R> Vbetahat <- vcov(thuesen.lm)
```

Given these quantities we can compute the vector **t** containing the two individual t test statistics and its associated correlation matrix as (see Section 3.1.1 for the theoretical background):

```
R> C <- diag(2)
R> Sigma <- diag(1 / sqrt(diag(C %*% Vbetahat %*% t(C))))
R> t <- Sigma %*% C %*% betahat
R> Cor <- Sigma %*% (C %*% Vbetahat %*% t(C)) %*% t(Sigma)
```

Note that $\mathbf{t} = (9.345, 2.101)^\top$ with associated correlation matrix

```
        [,1]    [,2]
[1,]   1.000 -0.923
[2,]  -0.923  1.000
```

Adjusted p-values are finally computed from the underlying bivariate t distribution using the pmvt function of the **mvtnorm** package (Hothorn, Bretz, and Genz 2001; Genz and Bretz 2009):

```
R> library("mvtnorm")
R> thuesen.df <- nrow(thuesen) - length(betahat)
R> q <- sapply(abs(t), function(x)
+              1 - pmvt(-rep(x, 2), rep(x, 2), corr = Cor,
+              df = thuesen.df))
```

We obtain the multiplicity adjusted p-values

$$q_1 < 0.001 \quad \text{and} \quad q_2 = 0.064, \tag{3.6}$$

indicating that the intercept is significantly different from 0 but the slope is not.

Alternatively, we can compute a critical value $u_{1-\alpha}$ derived from the bivariate t distribution and compare the test statistics $\mathbf{t} = (t_1, t_2)^\top$ against it. Using the function

```
R> delta <- rep(0, 2)
R> myfct <- function(x, conf) {
+      lower <- rep(-x, 2)
+      upper <- rep(x, 2)
+      pmvt(lower, upper, df = thuesen.df, corr = Cor,
+           delta, abseps = 0.0001)[1] - conf
+ }
```

we can compute the critical value $u_{1-\alpha}$ with the uniroot function

```
R> u <- uniroot(myfct, lower = 1, upper = 5, conf = 0.95)$root
R> round(u, 3)
```

```
[1] 2.23
```

In our example we set the confidence level as $1 - \alpha = 0.95$ and obtain $u_{1-\alpha} = 2.229$. Because the test statistics for the two-sided test problem are $|t_1| = 9.345 > u_{1-\alpha}$ and $|t_2| = 2.101 < u_{1-\alpha}$, we obtain the same test decisions as in (3.6). In addition, the critical value $u_{1-\alpha} = 2.229$ can be used to compute simultaneous confidence intervals for the parameters β_1 and β_2. Note that because the parameter estimates are highly correlated, the critical value 2.229 from the bivariate t distribution is considerably smaller than the Bonferroni critical value $t_{1-\alpha/2,\nu} = 2.414$ from the univariate t distribution.

As seen from the thuesen example, performing advanced multiple comparisons can involve a number of individual steps. The **multcomp** package provides a formal framework to replace the previous calculations with standardized function calls. Details of the **multcomp** package are given in Section 3.3, but for illustration purposes we apply it now to the thuesen data. The following lines replicate some of the calculations from Chapter 1, where we first used the **multcomp** package.

The glht function from **multcomp** takes a fitted response model and a matrix $\mathbf{C}$ defining the hypotheses of interest to perform the multiple comparisons:

```
R> library("multcomp")
R> thuesen.mc <- glht(thuesen.lm, linfct = C)
R> summary(thuesen.mc)
```

```
        Simultaneous Tests for General Linear Hypotheses

Fit: lm(formula = short.velocity ~ blood.glucose,
  data = thuesen)

Linear Hypotheses:
                   Estimate Std. Error t value Pr(>|t|)
(Intercept) == 0     1.0978     0.1175    9.34   1e-08 ***
blood.glucose == 0   0.0220     0.0105    2.10   0.064 .
---
Signif. codes:  0 '***' 0.001 '**' 0.01 '*' 0.05 '.' 0.1 ' ' 1
(Adjusted p values reported -- single-step method)
```

For each parameter $\beta_i, i = 1, 2$, **multcomp** reports its estimate and standard error. Taking the ratio of these two values for each parameter results in the reported test statistics. Adjusted p-values are given in the last column of the standard output from **multcomp**. As expected, they are the same as calculated in (3.6). In addition, simultaneous confidence intervals can be calculated for each parameter using the the `confint` method:

```
R> confint(thuesen.mc)
```

```
       Simultaneous Confidence Intervals

Fit: lm(formula = short.velocity ~ blood.glucose,
  data = thuesen)

Quantile = 2.23
95% family-wise confidence level


Linear Hypotheses:
                   Estimate lwr       upr
(Intercept) == 0    1.09781  0.83591   1.35972
blood.glucose == 0  0.02196 -0.00134   0.04527
```

The two-sided confidence interval for the slope includes the 0, thus reflecting the previous test decision that the slope is not statistically significant different from 0. We further conclude that the intercept lies roughly between 0.84 and 1.36.

So far we have only illustrated single-step procedures, which account for the correlation among the test statistics. As we know from Chapter 2, associated closed test procedures are available and uniformly more powerful. In **multcomp** we can call, for example,

```
R> summary(thuesen.mc, test = adjusted(type = "Westfall"))
            Simultaneous Tests for General Linear Hypotheses

Fit: lm(formula = short.velocity ~ blood.glucose,
   data = thuesen)

Linear Hypotheses:
                    Estimate Std. Error t value Pr(>|t|)
(Intercept) == 0      1.0978     0.1175    9.34   1e-08 ***
blood.glucose == 0    0.0220     0.0105    2.10   0.048 *
---
Signif. codes:  0 '***' 0.001 '**' 0.01 '*' 0.05 '.' 0.1 ' ' 1
(Adjusted p values reported -- Westfall method)
```

to extract related adjusted p-values. Note that the p-value associated with the slope parameter is now $p = 0.048 < 0.05$ and one can thus safely claim that the slope is significant at level $\alpha = 0.05$ after having adjusted for multiplicity. Details on the implemented stepwise procedures in the **multcomp** package are given in Section 3.3 and Chapter 4.

3.2 Extensions to general parametric models

In Section 3.1 we introduced multiple comparison procedures, which are well established for common regression and ANOVA models allowing for covariates and/or factorial treatment structures with independent and identically distributed normal errors and constant variance. In this section we extend these results and provide a unified description of multiple comparison procedures in parametric models with generally correlated parameter estimates. We relax the standard ANOVA assumptions, such as normality and homoscedasticity, thus allowing for simultaneous inference in generalized linear models, mixed-effects models, survival models, etc. As before, we assume that each individual null hypothesis is specified through a linear combination of p elemental model parameters and we simultaneously test m null hypotheses.

In Section 3.2.1 we introduce the necessary asymptotic results for the linear functions of interest under rather weak conditions. In Section 3.2.2 we describe the framework for multiple comparison procedures in general parametric models. We give important applications of the methodology in Section 3.2.3. Numerical examples to illustrate the methods using the **multcomp** package are left for Chapter 4. Much of the following material follows the outline of Hothorn, Bretz, and Westfall (2008).

3.2.1 Asymptotic results

We extend the notation from Section 3.1 to cope with the generality required below. Let $M(\{\mathbf{z}_1, \ldots, \mathbf{z}_n\}, \boldsymbol{\theta}, \boldsymbol{\eta})$ denote a parametric or semi-parametric statistical model, where $\{\mathbf{z}_1, \ldots, \mathbf{z}_n\}$ denotes the set of n observation vectors, $\boldsymbol{\theta}$ denotes the $p \times 1$ fixed parameter vector and the vector $\boldsymbol{\eta}$ contains other (random or nuisance) parameters. We are primarily interested in the linear functions $\boldsymbol{\vartheta} = \mathbf{C}^\top \boldsymbol{\theta}$ of the parameter vector $\boldsymbol{\theta}$ as specified through the $p \times m$ matrix $\mathbf{C}$ with fixed and known constants. Assume that we are given an estimate $\hat{\boldsymbol{\theta}}_n$ of the parameter vector $\boldsymbol{\theta}$. In what follows we describe the underlying model assumptions, the limiting distribution for the estimates of our parameters of interest, $\boldsymbol{\vartheta} = \mathbf{C}^\top \boldsymbol{\theta}$, as well as the corresponding test statistics for hypotheses involving $\boldsymbol{\vartheta}$ and their limiting joint distribution.

Consider, for example, a standard regression model to illustrate the new notation and how it relates to the one used in Section 3.1. Here, the observations $\mathbf{z}_i$ of subject $i = 1, \ldots, n$ consist of a response variable y_i and a vector of covariates $\mathbf{x}_i = (x_{i1}, \ldots, x_{ip})$, such that $\mathbf{z}_i = (y_i, \mathbf{x}_i)$ and $x_{i1} = 1$ for all i. The response is modeled by a linear combination of the covariates with normal error $\varepsilon_i \sim N(0, \sigma^2)$ and constant variance σ^2,

$$y_i = \beta_1 + \sum_{j=2}^{p} \beta_j x_{ij} + \varepsilon_i.$$

The parameter vector is then $\boldsymbol{\theta} = (\beta_1, \ldots, \beta_p)$, resulting in the linear functions of interest $\boldsymbol{\vartheta} = \mathbf{C}^\top \boldsymbol{\theta}$.

Coming back to the general theory, suppose $\hat{\boldsymbol{\theta}}_n$ is an estimate of $\boldsymbol{\theta}$ and $\mathbf{S}_n \in \mathbb{R}^{p,p}$ is an estimate of $\mathrm{cov}(\hat{\boldsymbol{\theta}}_n)$ with

$$a_n \mathbf{S}_n \xrightarrow{\mathbb{P}} \boldsymbol{\Sigma} \in \mathbb{R}^{p,p} \tag{3.7}$$

for some positive, nondecreasing sequence a_n. Furthermore, we assume that the multivariate central limit theorem holds, that is,

$$a_n^{1/2}(\hat{\boldsymbol{\theta}}_n - \boldsymbol{\theta}) \xrightarrow{d} N_p(0, \boldsymbol{\Sigma}). \tag{3.8}$$

If both (3.7) and (3.8) are fulfilled, we write $\hat{\boldsymbol{\theta}}_n \overset{a}{\sim} N_p(\boldsymbol{\theta}, \mathbf{S}_n)$. Then, by Theorem 3.3.A in Serfling (1980), the estimate of our parameter of interest, $\hat{\boldsymbol{\vartheta}}_n = \mathbf{C}^\top \hat{\boldsymbol{\theta}}_n$, is approximately multivariate normally distributed, that is,

$$\hat{\boldsymbol{\vartheta}}_n = \mathbf{C}^\top \hat{\boldsymbol{\theta}}_n \overset{a}{\sim} N_m(\boldsymbol{\vartheta}, \mathbf{S}_n^\star)$$

with covariance matrix $\mathbf{S}_n^\star = \mathbf{C}^\top \mathbf{S}_n \mathbf{C}$ for any fixed matrix $\mathbf{C}$. Thus, we do not need to distinguish between the model parameter $\boldsymbol{\theta}$ and the derived parameter $\boldsymbol{\vartheta} = \mathbf{C}^\top \boldsymbol{\theta}$. In analogy to (3.7) and (3.8) we can thus assume that

$$\hat{\boldsymbol{\vartheta}}_n \overset{a}{\sim} N_m(\boldsymbol{\vartheta}, \mathbf{S}_n^\star)$$

holds, where

$$a_n \mathbf{S}_n^\star \xrightarrow{\mathbb{P}} \boldsymbol{\Sigma}^\star = \mathbf{C}^\top \boldsymbol{\Sigma} \mathbf{C} \in \mathbb{R}^{m,m},$$

and that the m parameters in $\boldsymbol{\vartheta}$ are the parameters of interest. It is assumed that the diagonal elements of the covariance matrix are positive, that is, $\Sigma_{jj}^\star > 0$ for $j = 1, \ldots, m$. Consequently, the standardized estimate $\hat{\boldsymbol{\vartheta}}_n$ is again asymptotically multivariate normally distributed. Following Hothorn et al. (2008),

$$\mathbf{t}_n = \mathbf{D}_n^{-1/2}(\hat{\boldsymbol{\vartheta}}_n - \boldsymbol{\vartheta}) \overset{a}{\sim} N_m(0, \mathbf{R}_n)$$

where $\mathbf{D}_n = \mathrm{diag}(\mathbf{S}_n^\star)$ contains the diagonal elements of $\mathbf{S}_n^\star$ and

$$\mathbf{R}_n = \mathbf{D}_n^{-1/2}\mathbf{S}_n^\star\mathbf{D}_n^{-1/2} \in \mathbb{R}^{m,m}$$

is the correlation matrix of the m-dimensional statistic $\mathbf{t}_n$. This leads to the main asymptotic result in this section,

$$\mathbf{t}_n = (a_n\mathbf{D}_n)^{-1/2}a_n^{1/2}(\hat{\boldsymbol{\vartheta}}_n - \boldsymbol{\vartheta}) \xrightarrow{d} N_m(\mathbf{0}, \mathbf{R}).$$

For the purpose of multiple comparisons, we need convergence of multivariate probabilities calculated for the vector $\mathbf{t}_n$, where $\mathbf{t}_n$ is assumed normally distributed and $\mathbf{R}_n$ treated as if it was the true correlation matrix. However, the necessary probabilities are continuous functions of $\mathbf{R}_n$ (and the associated critical value) which converge by $\mathbf{R}_n \xrightarrow{\mathbb{P}} \mathbf{R}$ as a consequence of Theorem 1.7 in Serfling (1980). In cases where $\mathbf{t}_n$ is assumed to be multivariate t distributed with $\mathbf{R}_n$ treated as the estimated correlation matrix, we have similar convergence as the degrees of freedom approach infinity.

Since we only assume that the parameter estimates $\hat{\boldsymbol{\theta}}_n$ are asymptotically normally distributed with an available consistent estimate of the associated covariance matrix, the framework in this section covers a wide range of statistical models, including linear regression and ANOVA models, generalized linear models, linear mixed-effects models, Cox models, robust linear models, etc. Standard software packages can be used to fit such models and obtain the estimates $\hat{\boldsymbol{\theta}}_n$ and $\mathbf{S}_n$, which are the only two quantities that are needed here.

3.2.2 Multiple comparisons in general parametric models

Based on the asymptotic results from Section 3.2.1, we can derive suitable multiple comparison procedures for the class of parametric models introduced there. We start considering the global null hypothesis

$$H: \boldsymbol{\vartheta} = \mathbf{a}$$

where, as before, $\boldsymbol{\vartheta} = \mathbf{C}^\top\boldsymbol{\theta}$ and $\mathbf{a} = (a_1, \ldots, a_m)^\top$ denotes a vector of fixed and known constants. Under the conditions of H it follows from Section 3.2.1 that

$$\mathbf{t}_n = \mathbf{D}_n^{-1/2}(\hat{\boldsymbol{\vartheta}}_n - \mathbf{a}) \overset{a}{\sim} N_m(\mathbf{0}, \mathbf{R}_n).$$

This approximating distribution will be used as the reference distribution when constructing suitable multiple comparison procedures below. Note that the asymptotic results can be sharpened if we assume exact normality $\hat{\boldsymbol{\theta}}_n \sim N_p(\boldsymbol{\theta}, \boldsymbol{\Sigma})$ instead of the asymptotic normality assumption (3.8). If the covariance matrix $\boldsymbol{\Sigma}$ is known, it follows by standard arguments that $\mathbf{t}_n \sim N_m(\mathbf{0}, \mathbf{R})$, where $\mathbf{t}_n$ is normalized using fixed and known variances. Otherwise, in the typical situation of linear models with independent, normally distributed errors and $\boldsymbol{\Sigma} = \sigma^2\mathbf{A}$, where σ^2 is unknown but $\mathbf{A}$ is fixed and known, the exact distribution of $\mathbf{t}_n$ is multivariate t; see Section 3.1.1.

The global null hypothesis H can be tested using standard tests, such as F or χ^2 tests, see Hothorn et al. (2008) for analytical expressions. An alternative approach is to consider the maximum of the individual components of the vector $\mathbf{t}_n = (t_{1n}, \ldots, t_{mn})$, leading to the max-$t$ test $t_{\max} = \max |\mathbf{t}_n|$ (see also Section 2.2.1 for a brief discussion about max-t tests). The distribution of this statistic under the conditions of H can be computed using the m-dimensional distribution function

$$\mathbb{P}(t_{\max} \leq t) \cong \int_{-t}^{t} \cdots \int_{-t}^{t} \varphi_m(\mathbf{x}; \mathbf{R}, \nu)d\mathbf{x} =: g_\nu(\mathbf{R}, t) \tag{3.9}$$

for some $t \in \mathbb{R}$, where φ_m denotes the density function of either the limiting m-dimensional normal (with $\nu = \infty$ degrees of freedom and the "$\approx$" operator) or the exact multivariate t distribution (with $\nu < \infty$ and the "$=$" operator). Because $\mathbf{R}$ is usually unknown, we plug in the consistent estimate $\mathbf{R}_n$, as discussed in Section 3.2.1. The resulting (exact or asymptotic) p-value for H is then given by $1 - g_\nu(\mathbf{R}_n, \max |\mathbf{t}^{\text{obs}}|)$, where $\mathbf{t}^{\text{obs}} = (t_1^{\text{obs}}, \ldots, t_m^{\text{obs}})$ denotes the vector of observed test statistics t_j^{obs}. Efficient methods to calculate multivariate normal and t integrals are described in Genz and Bretz (1999, 2002, 2009).

Note that in contrast to standard global F or χ^2 tests, max-t tests of the form $t_{\max} = \max |\mathbf{t}_n|$ additionally provide information about the elementary null hypotheses (consonance property, see Section 2.2.1). To this end, recall that $\mathbf{C} = (\mathbf{c}_1, \ldots, \mathbf{c}_m)$ and let $\vartheta_j = \mathbf{c}_j^\top \boldsymbol{\theta}$ denote the j-th linear function of interest, $j = 1, \ldots, m$. The elementary null hypotheses of interest are given by

$$H_j : \mathbf{c}_j^\top \boldsymbol{\theta} = a_j, \quad j = 1, \ldots, m,$$

for fixed and known constants a_j, such that $H = \bigcap_{j=1}^m H_j$. Adjusted p-values (exact or asymptotic) are given by

$$q_j = 1 - g_\nu(\mathbf{R}_n, |t_j^{\text{obs}}|), \quad j = 1, \ldots, m,$$

and calculated from expression (3.9). By construction, we reject an elementary null hypothesis H_j whenever the associated adjusted p-value q_j is less than or equal to the pre-specified significance level α, that is, $q_j \leq \alpha$. Alternatively, if $u_{1-\alpha}$ denotes the $(1-\alpha)$-quantile of the distribution (asymptotic, if necessary) of $\mathbf{t}_n$, we reject H_j if $|t_j^{\text{obs}}| \geq u_{1-\alpha}$. In addition, simultaneous confidence intervals for ϑ_j with coverage probability $1 - \alpha$ can be constructed from $\hat{\vartheta}_n \pm u_{1-\alpha}\text{diag}(\mathbf{D}_n)^{1/2}$. Similar results also hold for one-sided test problems.

Similar to Section 3.1.1, the methods discussed here can be used to construct more powerful closed test procedures, as first discussed by Westfall (1997). That is, applying closed test procedures (Section 2.2.3) based on max-t tests of the form (2.1) in combination with the results from here gives powerful stepwise procedures for a large class of parametric models. The **multcomp** package implements these methods while exploiting logical constraints, leading to computationally efficient, yet powerful truncated closed test procedures (Westfall and Tobias 2007), as described in Section 3.3 and illustrated with examples in Chapter 4.

3.2.3 Applications

The methodological framework described in Section 3.2.1 is very general and thus applicable to a wide range of statistical models. Many estimation techniques, such as (restricted) maximum likelihood and M estimates, provide at least asymptotical normal estimates of the original parameter vector $\boldsymbol{\theta}$ and a consistent estimate of the covariance matrix. In this section we review some potential applications. Detailed numerical examples are discussed in Chapter 4.

In Section 3.2.1 we already provided a connection between the general parametric framework and standard *regression* models. Similarly, *ANOVA models* are easily embedded in that framework as well. With an appropriate change of notation, one can verify that the results from Section 3.1 are a special case of the general framework considered in Section 3.2.1.

In *generalized linear models*, the exact distribution of the parameter estimates is usually unknown and the asymptotic normal distribution is the basis for all inference procedures. If inferences about model parameters corresponding to levels of a certain factor are of interest, one can use the multiple comparison procedures described above.

Similarly, in linear and non-linear mixed-effects models fitted by restricted maximum likelihood, the asymptotic normal distribution using consistent covariance matrix estimates forms the basis for inference. All assumptions of the general parametric framework are satisfied again and one can set up simultaneous inference procedures for these models as well. The same is true for either the *Cox model* or other parametric survival models such as the *Weibull survival model*.

Yet another application is to use robust variants of the previously discussed statistical models. One possibility is to consider the use of sandwich estimators S_n for the covariance matrix $\operatorname{cov}(\boldsymbol{\theta}_n)$ when the variance homogeneity assumption is questionable. An alternative approach is to apply robust estimation techniques in linear models (such as S-, M- or MM-estimates), which again provide asymptotically normal estimates (Rousseeuw and Leroy 2003).

Herberich (2009) investigated through an extensive simulation study the operating characteristics (size and power) of the multiple comparison procedures described in this section for a variety of statistical models (generalized linear models, mixed effects models, survival data, etc.). It transpires that the family-wise error rate is generally well maintained even for moderate to small sample sizes, although under certain models and scenarios the resulting tests may become either conservative (especially for binary data with small sample sizes) or liberal (survival data, depending on the censoring mechanism). Further simulations indicated a good overall performance of the proposed parametric multiple comparison procedures compared with existing procedures, such as the simultaneous confidence intervals for binomial parameters introduced by Agresti, Bini, Bertaccini, and Ryu (2008).

3.3 The multcomp package

In this section we introduce the **multcomp** package in R to perform multiple comparisons under the parametric model framework described in Sections 3.1 and 3.2. In Section 3.3.1 we detail the `glht` function, which provides the core functionality to perform single-step tests based on a given matrix $\mathbf{C}$ reflecting the experimental questions of interest and the underlying multivariate normal or t distribution. In Section 3.3.2 we describe the `summary` method associated with the `glht` function, which provides detailed output information, including the results of several p-value adjustment methods and stepwise test procedures. Finally, we describe in Section 3.3.3 the `confint` method associated with the `glht` function, which provides the functionality to compute and plot simultaneous confidence intervals for some of the multiple comparison procedures. The **multcomp** package includes additional functionality not covered in this section. In Chapter 4 we illustrate some of its enhanced capabilities. The complete documentation is available with the package (Hothorn, Bretz, Westfall, Heiberger, and Schützenmeister 2010a). As any other package used in this book, the **multcomp** package can be downloaded from CRAN.

3.3.1 The glht function

In this section we consider the `warpbreaks` data from Tukey (1977), which are also available from the base R **datasets** package. The data give the number of breaks in yarn during weaving for two types of wool (A and B) and three levels of tension (L, M, and H). For illustration purposes, here we only consider the effect of the tension on the number of breaks, neglecting the potential effect of the wool type. Figure 3.1 shows the associated boxplots for the data.

Assume that we are interested in assessing whether the three levels of tension differ from each other with respect to the number of breaks. In other words, if μ_j denotes the mean number of breaks for tension level $j = L, M, H$, we are interested in testing the three null hypotheses

$$H_{ij} : \mu_i - \mu_j = 0 \qquad (3.10)$$

against the alternative hypotheses

$$K_{ij} : \mu_i - \mu_j \neq 0, \quad i, j \in \{L, M, H, \}, i \neq j.$$

In the following we use this example to illustrate the **multcomp** package. To analyze the `warpbreaks` data we use the well-known Tukey test, which perfoms all pairwise comparisons between the three treatments and which we formally introduce in Section 4.2. We use the `aov` function to fit the one-factor ANOVA model

```
R> warpbreaks.aov <- aov(breaks ~ tension, data = warpbreaks)
R> summary(warpbreaks.aov)

           Df Sum Sq Mean Sq F value Pr(>F)
tension     2   2034    1017    7.21 0.0018 **
```

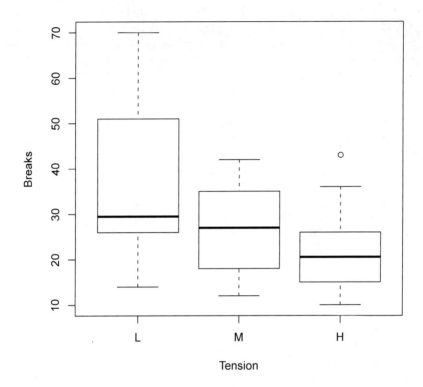

Figure 3.1   Boxplots of the `warpbreaks` data.

```
Residuals    51    7199       141
---
Signif. codes:   0 '***' 0.001 '**' 0.01 '*' 0.05 '.' 0.1 ' ' 1
```

Based on the ANOVA F test we conclude that the factor `tension` has an overall significant effect.

The `glht` function from the **multcomp** package provides a convenient and general framework in R to test multiple hypotheses in parametric models, including the general linear models introduced in Section 3.1, linear and non-linear mixed-effects models as well as survival models. Generally speaking, the `glht` function takes a fitted response model and a matrix **C** defining the hypotheses of interest to perform the multiple comparisons. The general syntax for the `glht` function is

```
glht(model,
     linfct,
     alternative = c("two.sided", "less", "greater"),
     rhs = 0,
     ...
)
```

In this call, the `model` argument is a fitted model, such as an object returned by `lm`, `glm`, or `aov`. It is assumed that the parameter estimates and their covariance matrix are available for the `model` argument. That is, the `model` argument needs suitable `coef` and `vcov` methods to be available. The argument `linfct` specifies the matrix **C** introduced in Section 3.1. There are alternative ways of specifying the matrix **C** and we illustrate them below using the `warpbreaks` example. The `alternative` argument is a character string specifying the alternative hypothesis, which must be one of `"two.sided"` (default), `"greater"` or `"less"`, depending on whether two-sided or one-sided hypotheses are of interest. The `rhs` argument is an optional numeric vector specifying the right hand side of the hypothesis (in Equation (3.10) the right hand side is 0 for all three hypotheses). Finally, with "..." additional arguments can be passed on to the `modelparm` function in all `glht` methods.

We now review the different possibilities of specifying the matrix **C**, which can, but does not have to be a contrast matrix; see Section 3.1.1 for the definition of a contrast. The most convenient way is to use the `mcp` function. Multiple comparisons of means are defined by objects of the `mcp` class as returned by the `mcp` function. For each factor contained in `model` as an independent variable, a (contrast) matrix or a symbolic description of the comparisons of interest can be specified as an argument to `mcp`. A symbolic description may be a `character` or an `expression` where the factor levels are only used as variables names. In addition, the `type` argument to the (contrast) matrix generating function `contrMat` may serve as a symbolic description as well. To illustrate the latter, we invoke the Tukey test consisting of all pairwise comparisons for the factor `tension` by using a symbolic description, that is, using the `type` argument to the `contrMat` function

```
R> glht(warpbreaks.aov, linfct = mcp(tension = "Tukey"))

         General Linear Hypotheses

Multiple Comparisons of Means: Tukey Contrasts


Linear Hypotheses:
           Estimate
M - L == 0   -10.00
H - L == 0   -14.72
H - M == 0    -4.72
```

Note that the `contrMat` function also permits pre-specifying other contrast matrices, such as `"Dunnett"`, `"Williams"`, and `"Changepoint"`; see Section 4.3.2

for further examples and the online documentation for a complete list (Hothorn et al. 2010a).

Another way of defining the matrix $\mathbf{C}$ is to use a symbolic description, where either a `character` or an `expression` vector is passed to `glht` via its `linfct` argument. A symbolic description must be interpretable as a valid R expression consisting of both the left and the right hand side of the expression for the null hypotheses. Only the names of `coef(beta)` can be used as variable names. The alternative hypotheses are given by the direction under the null hypothesis (= or == refer to `"two.sided"`, <= refers to `"greater"` and >= refers to `"less"`). Numeric vectors of length one are valid arguments for the right hand side. If we call

```
R> glht(warpbreaks.aov,
+        linfct = mcp(tension = c("M - L = 0",
+                                 "H - L = 0",
+                                 "H - M = 0")))
```

```
            General Linear Hypotheses

Multiple Comparisons of Means: User-defined Contrasts


Linear Hypotheses:
            Estimate
M - L == 0    -10.00
H - L == 0    -14.72
H - M == 0     -4.72
```

we obtain the same results as before.

Alternatively, the matrix $\mathbf{C}$ can be defined directly by calling

```
R> contr <- rbind("M - L" = c(-1,  1, 0),
+                 "H - L" = c(-1,  0, 1),
+                 "H - M" = c( 0, -1, 1))
R> contr
```

```
        [,1] [,2] [,3]
M - L     -1    1    0
H - L     -1    0    1
H - M      0   -1    1
```

and again we obtain the same results as before:

```
R> glht(warpbreaks.aov, linfct = mcp(tension = contr))
            General Linear Hypotheses

Multiple Comparisons of Means: User-defined Contrasts


Linear Hypotheses:
            Estimate
```

```
M - L == 0    -10.00
H - L == 0    -14.72
H - M == 0     -4.72
```

Finally, the matrix **C** can be specified directly via the `linfct` argument. In this case, the number of columns of the matrix needs to match the number of parameters estimated by `model`. It is assumed that suitable `coef` and `vcov` methods are available for `model`. In the `warpbreaks` example, we can specify

```
R> glht(warpbreaks.aov,
+          linfct = cbind(0, contr %*% contr.treatment(3)))
```

General Linear Hypotheses

```
Linear Hypotheses:
              Estimate
M - L == 0    -10.00
H - L == 0    -14.72
H - M == 0     -4.72
```

and again we obtain the same results as before. Note that in the last statement we used the so-called *treatment contrasts*

```
R> contr.treatment(3)
```

```
  2 3
1 0 0
2 1 0
3 0 1
```

which are used as default in R to fit ANOVA and regression models. The first group is treated as a control group, to which the other groups are compared. To be more specific, the analysis is performed as a multiple regression analysis by introducing two dummy variables which are 1 for observations in the relevant group and 0 elsewhere.

We now turn our attention to the description of the output from the `glht` function and the available methods for further analyses. Using the `glht` function, a list is returned with the elements

```
R> warpbreaks.mc <- glht(warpbreaks.aov,
+                        linfct = mcp(tension = "Tukey"))
R> names(warpbreaks.mc)
```

```
[1] "model"       "linfct"      "rhs"         "coef"
[5] "vcov"        "df"          "alternative" "type"
[9] "focus"
```

where `print`, `summary`, and `confint` methods are available for further information handling. If `glht` is called with `linfct` as an `mcp` object, the additional element `focus` is available, which stores the names of the factors tested. In the following we describe the output in more detail. Some of the associated methods will be discussed in the subsequent sections.

The first element of the returned object

```
R> warpbreaks.mc$model
```

```
Call:
   aov(formula = breaks ~ tension, data = warpbreaks)

Terms:
                 tension Residuals
Sum of Squares      2034      7199
Deg. of Freedom        2        51

Residual standard error: 11.9
Estimated effects may be unbalanced
```

gives the fitted model, as used in the `glht` call. The element

```
R> warpbreaks.mc$linfct
```

```
      (Intercept) tensionM tensionH
M - L           0        1        0
H - L           0        0        1
H - M           0       -1        1
attr(,"type")
[1] "Tukey"
```

returns the matrix $\mathbf{C}$ used for the definition of the linear functions of interest, as discussed above. Each row of this matrix essentially defines the left hand side of the hypotheses defined in equation (3.2). The associated right hand side of equation (3.2) is returned by

```
R> warpbreaks.mc$rhs
```

```
[1] 0 0 0
```

The next two elements of the list returned by the `glht` function give the estimates and the associated covariance matrix of the parameters specified through `model`,

```
R> warpbreaks.mc$coef
```

```
(Intercept)      tensionM      tensionH
      36.4         -10.0         -14.7
```

```
R> warpbreaks.mc$vcov
```

```
             (Intercept) tensionM tensionH
(Intercept)         7.84    -7.84    -7.84
tensionM           -7.84    15.68     7.84
tensionH           -7.84     7.84    15.68
```

As an optional element the degrees of freedom

```
R> warpbreaks.mc$df
```

```
[1] 51
```

is returned if the multivariate t distribution is used for simultaneous inference. Because we have 54 observations in total for the `warpbreaks` data and the factor `tension` has 3 levels, we obtain the displayed 51 degrees of freedom for the underlying one-way layout. Note that inference is based on the multivariate t distribution whenever a linear model with normally distributed errors is applied; the limiting multivariate normal distribution is used in all other cases. The element

```
R> warpbreaks.mc$alternative
```

```
[1] "two.sided"
```

is a character string specifying the sideness of the test problem. Finally,

```
R> warpbreaks.mc$type
```

```
[1] "Tukey"
```

optionally specifies the name of the applied multiple comparison procedure.

3.3.2 The *summary* method

The **multcomp** package provides a `summary` method to summarize and display the results returned from the `glht` function. In addition, the `summary` method provides several functionalities to perform further analyses and adjustments for multiplicity. We start applying the `summary` method to the object returned by `glht` as

```
R> summary(warpbreaks.mc)

        Simultaneous Tests for General Linear Hypotheses

Multiple Comparisons of Means: Tukey Contrasts


Fit: aov(formula = breaks ~ tension, data = warpbreaks)

Linear Hypotheses:
             Estimate Std. Error t value Pr(>|t|)
M - L == 0     -10.00       3.96   -2.53   0.0385 *
H - L == 0     -14.72       3.96   -3.72   0.0014 **
H - M == 0      -4.72       3.96   -1.19   0.4631
---
Signif. codes:  0 '***' 0.001 '**' 0.01 '*' 0.05 '.' 0.1 ' ' 1
(Adjusted p values reported -- single-step method)
```

As seen from the output above, for each of the $m = 3$ linear functions of interest the estimates $\mathbf{c}_j^\top \hat{\boldsymbol{\beta}}$ are reported together with the associated standard errors $\sqrt{\hat{\mathbb{V}}(\mathbf{c}_j^\top \hat{\boldsymbol{\beta}})}$, resulting in the test statistics

$$ t_j = \frac{\mathbf{c}_j^\top \hat{\boldsymbol{\beta}}}{\sqrt{\hat{\mathbb{V}}(\mathbf{c}_j^\top \hat{\boldsymbol{\beta}})}}, \quad j = 1, 2, 3, $$

recall Equation (3.5) for the general expression (note that $\mathbf{a} = \mathbf{0}$ in the warpbreaks example). Multiplicity adjusted p-values q_j are reported in the last column. These p-values are calculated from the underlying multivariate t (or normal, if appropriate) distribution and can be directly compared with the significance level α. In the warpbreaks example, we conclude that both tension levels M (medium) and H (high) are significantly different from L (low) at level $\alpha = 0.05$, because $q_1 = q_{ML} = 0.0385 < 0.05 = \alpha$ and $q_2 = q_{HL} = 0.0014 < 0.05$. Note that $q_3 = q_{HM} = 0.4631 > 0.05$ and the tension levels M and H are not declared to be significantly different.

If we save the information provided by the summary method into the object

```
R> warpbreaks.res <- summary(warpbreaks.mc)
```

we can extract the numerical information from the resulting list element warpbreaks.res$test for further analyses. For example,

```
R> warpbreaks.res$test$pvalues
[1] 0.03840 0.00144 0.46307
attr(, "error")
[1] 0.000184
```

returns the adjusted p-values from the previous analysis.

In addition to summarizing and displaying the information from the object returned by the glht function, the summary method provides a test argument, which allows one to peform further analyses. Recall Equation (3.10) for the elementary null hypotheses of interest in the warpbreaks example. The global null hypothesis $H = H_{ML} \cap H_{HL} \cap H_{HM}$ can then be tested with the common F test by calling

```
R> summary(warpbreaks.mc, test = Ftest())

        General Linear Hypotheses

Multiple Comparisons of Means: Tukey Contrasts


Linear Hypotheses:
           Estimate
M - L == 0   -10.00
H - L == 0   -14.72
H - M == 0    -4.72

Global Test:
    F DF1 DF2  Pr(>F)
1 7.2   2  51 0.00175
```

Note that the above F test result coincides with the result from the analysis following Equation (3.10), where we used the aov function to fit the one-factor ANOVA model. Similarly, a Wald test can be performed by specifying Chisqtest().

If no multiplicity adjustment is foreseen, the univariate() option can be passed to the test argument

```
R> summary(warpbreaks.mc, test = univariate())
```

```
         Simultaneous Tests for General Linear Hypotheses

Multiple Comparisons of Means: Tukey Contrasts


Fit: aov(formula = breaks ~ tension, data = warpbreaks)

Linear Hypotheses:
          Estimate Std. Error t value Pr(>|t|)
M - L == 0   -10.00       3.96   -2.53   0.0147 *
H - L == 0   -14.72       3.96   -3.72   0.0005 ***
H - M == 0    -4.72       3.96   -1.19   0.2386
---
Signif. codes:  0 '***' 0.001 '**' 0.01 '*' 0.05 '.' 0.1 ' ' 1
(Univariate p values reported)
```

This results in unadjusted p-values, as if we had performed m separate t tests without accounting for multiplicity. If we compare the unadjusted p-values p_j from the output above with the adjusted p-values q_j from the Tukey test, we conclude that $p_j < q_j, j = 1, 2, 3$, as expected.

Table 3.1 summarizes the multiplicity adjustment methods available with the summary method via the adjusted argument to the test function. In particular, an interface to the multiplicity adjustments implemented in the p.adjust function from the **stats** package is available. Given a set of unadjusted p-values, the p.adjust function provides the resulting adjusted p-values using one of several methods. Currently, the following methods implemented in p.adjust are available: "none" (no multiplicity adjustment), "bonferroni" (Section 2.3.1), "holm" (Section 2.3.2), "hochberg" (Section 2.4), "hommel" (Section 2.4), "BH" (Benjamini and Hochberg 1995), and "BY" (Benjamini and Yekutieli 2001). The last two methods are tailored to control the false discovery rate; see Section 2.1.1. To illustrate the functionality, assume that we want to apply the Bonferroni correction to the warpbreaks data. This can be achieved by specifying the type argument to the adjusted option as

```
R> summary(warpbreaks.mc, test = adjusted(type = "bonferroni"))
         Simultaneous Tests for General Linear Hypotheses

Multiple Comparisons of Means: Tukey Contrasts


Fit: aov(formula = breaks ~ tension, data = warpbreaks)

Linear Hypotheses:
          Estimate Std. Error t value Pr(>|t|)
M - L == 0   -10.00       3.96   -2.53   0.0442 *
H - L == 0   -14.72       3.96   -3.72   0.0015 **
H - M == 0    -4.72       3.96   -1.19   0.7158
```

type argument to adjusted	Reference (section number)	Comments
"none"		no multiplicity adjustment; identical to test=univariate() option
"BH", "BY"		procedures controlling the false discovery rate
"bonferroni"	2.3.1	
"holm"	2.3.2	stepwise extension of and more powerful than "bonferroni"
"hochberg"	2.4	based on Simes test; more powerful than "holm", but has additional assumptions
"hommel"	2.4	more powerful than "hochberg"
"single-step"	3.1, 3.2	default option; incorporates correlations and is more powerful than "bonferroni"
"free"	4.1.2	stepwise extension of and more powerful than "single-step"
"Shaffer"	2.3.2	stepwise extension of "bonferroni" under restricted combination condition
"Westfall"	4.2.2	extension of "Shaffer" that incorporates correlations

Table 3.1 Multiple comparison procedures available with the **summary** method from the **multcomp** package. In addition, global F and χ^2 tests are available as direct arguments to **test**.

```
---
Signif. codes:  0 '***' 0.001 '**' 0.01 '*' 0.05 '.' 0.1 ' ' 1
(Adjusted p values reported -- bonferroni method)
```

Note that all methods from the `p.adjust` function are based on unadjusted p-values. More powerful methods are available by taking the correlations between the test statistics into account, as described in Sections 3.1 and 3.2. In **multcomp**, four additional options for the `type` argument to `adjusted` are implemented to accomplish this. The `type = "single-step"` option specifies a single-step test (Section 2.1.2), which incorporates the correlations between the test statistics using either the multivariate normal or t distribution implemented in the **mvtnorm** package (Genz, Bretz, and Hothorn 2010). Consequently, calling

```
R> summary(warpbreaks.mc, test = adjusted(type = "single-step"))
```

```
        Simultaneous Tests for General Linear Hypotheses

Multiple Comparisons of Means: Tukey Contrasts


Fit: aov(formula = breaks ~ tension, data = warpbreaks)

Linear Hypotheses:
            Estimate Std. Error t value Pr(>|t|)
M - L == 0    -10.00       3.96   -2.53   0.0385 *
H - L == 0    -14.72       3.96   -3.72   0.0014 **
H - M == 0     -4.72       3.96   -1.19   0.4631
---
Signif. codes:  0 '***' 0.001 '**' 0.01 '*' 0.05 '.' 0.1 ' ' 1
(Adjusted p values reported -- single-step method)
```

results in the same adjusted p-values and test decisions as for the Tukey test considered previously. The `type = "free"` option leads to a step-down test procedure under the free combination condition (Section 2.1.2), which incorporates correlations and is thus more powerful than the Holm procedure; see Section 4.1.2 for a detailed description of its usage. Under the restricted combination condition, the `type = "Shaffer"` option performs the $S2$ procedure from Shaffer (1986), which uses Bonferroni tests for each intersection hypothesis of the underlying closed test procedure (Section 2.3.2). When the tests satisfy the free combinations condition instead, Shaffer's procedure reduces to the ordinary Holm procedure. Finally, `type = "Westfall"` is yet more powerful than Shaffer's procedure. The increase in power comes from using specific dependence information rather than the conservative Bonferroni inequality (Westfall 1997; Westfall and Tobias 2007); see Section 4.2.2 for a detailed discussion.

3.3.3 The `confint` method

So far we have focused on the capabilities of **multcomp** to provide adjusted p-values for a variety of multiple comparison procedures. In this section we describe the available functionality to compute and plot simultaneous confidence intervals using the `confint` method. As mentioned in Section 2.1.2, simultaneous confidence intervals are available in closed form for many standard single-step procedures, but they are usually more difficult to derive for stepwise procedures. Consequently, the `confint` method implements simultaneous confidence intervals for single-step tests in the parametric model framework from Sections 3.1 and 3.2. Note that the `confint` method is only available for `glht` objects. Simultaneous confidence intervals for the Bonferroni test, for example, are not directly available but can be computed by specifying the `calpha` argument; see further below.

Consider again the `warpbreaks` example analyzed previously in this chapter. We can calculate simultaneous confidence intervals for the Tukey test by applying the `confint` method to the `warpbreaks.mc` object from the `glht` function:

```
R> warpbreaks.ci <- confint(warpbreaks.mc, level = 0.95)
R> warpbreaks.ci

        Simultaneous Confidence Intervals

Multiple Comparisons of Means: Tukey Contrasts


Fit: aov(formula = breaks ~ tension, data = warpbreaks)

Quantile = 2.41
95% family-wise confidence level


Linear Hypotheses:
           Estimate lwr      upr
M - L == 0 -10.000  -19.559  -0.441
H - L == 0 -14.722  -24.281  -5.164
H - M == 0  -4.722  -14.281   4.836
```

We conclude from the output that the upper confidence bounds for the pairwise differences $\mu_M - \mu_L$ and $\mu_H - \mu_L$ are negative, indicating that both tension levels M (medium) and H (high) significantly reduce the number of breaks as compared to tension level L (low). Moreover, we cannot conclude at the 95% confidence level that the groups M and H differ significantly. In addition, we can display the confidence intervals graphically using the associated `plot` method

```
R> plot(warpbreaks.ci, main = "", ylim = c(0.5, 3.5),
+        xlab = "Breaks")
```

see Figure 3.2 for the resulting plot. An improved greaphical display of the confidence intervals is available with the `plot.matchMMC` command from the **HH** package (Heiberger 2009); see Section 4.2.1 for an example of its use.

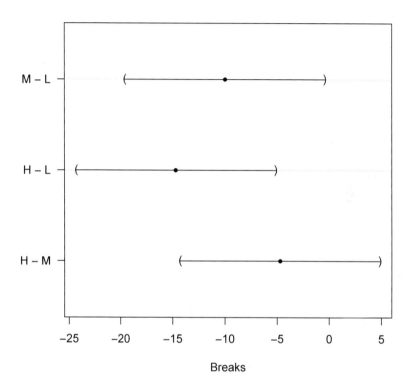

Figure 3.2   Two-sided simultaneous confidence intervals for the Tukey test in the `warpbreaks` example.

Note that unadjusted (marginal) confidence intervals can be computed by specifying `calpha = univariate_calpha()` to `confint`. Alternatively, the critical value can be directly specified as a scalar to `calpha`. In the previous example, the 95% critical value $u_{0.95} = 2.4142$ was calculated from the multivariate t distribution using the **mvtnorm** package. If instead

```
R> cbon <- qt(1-0.05/6, 51)
R> cbon
```

[1] 2.48

was specified to `calpha`, one would obtain the two-sided 95% simultaneous confidence intervals for the Bonferroni test with

```
R> confint(warpbreaks.mc, calpha = cbon)

        Simultaneous Confidence Intervals

Multiple Comparisons of Means: Tukey Contrasts


Fit: aov(formula = breaks ~ tension, data = warpbreaks)

Quantile = 2.48
95% confidence level


Linear Hypotheses:
          Estimate lwr       upr
M - L == 0 -10.000  -19.804   -0.196
H - L == 0 -14.722  -24.526   -4.919
H - M == 0  -4.722  -14.526    5.081
```

In case of all pairwise comparisons among several treatments, the **mult-comp** package also provides the option of plotting the results using a *compact letter display* (Piepho 2004). With this display, treatments that are not significantly different are assigned a common letter. In other words, significantly different treatments have no letters in common. This type of graphical display has advantages when a large number of treatments is being compared with each other, as it summarizes the test results more efficiently than a simple collection of simultaneous confidence intervals.

Using **multcomp**, the cld function extracts the necessary information from glht, summary.glht or confint.glht objects to create a compact letter display of all pairwise comparisons. In case of confint.glht objects, a pairwise comparison is reported significant if the associated simultaneous confidence interval does not contain 0. Otherwise, the associated adjusted p-value is compared with the given significance level α. For the warpbreaks example, we can extract the necessary information from the glht object by calling

```
R> warpbreaks.cld <- cld(warpbreaks.mc)
```

Once this information has been extracted, we can use a plot method associated with cld objects to create the compact letter display of all pairwise comparisons. If the fitted model contains any covariates, boxplots for each level are plotted. Otherwise, different types of plots are used, depending on the class of the response variable and the cld object; see the online documentation for further details (Hothorn et al. 2010a).

Figure 3.3 reproduces the boxplots for each of the three tension levels from Figure 3.1 together with the letter display when using the command

```
R> plot(warpbreaks.cld)
```

Because tension level L has no letter in common with any other tension level, it is significantly different at the chosen significance level ($\alpha = 0.05$ by default).

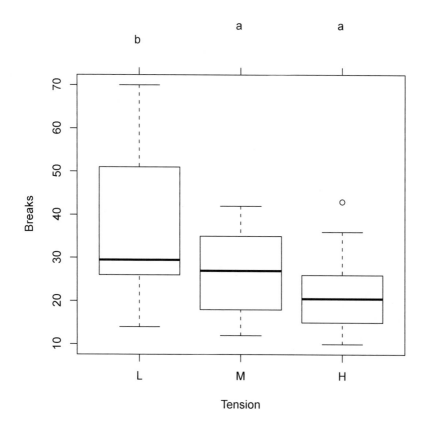

Figure 3.3 Compact letter display for all pairwise comparisons in the `warpbreaks` example.

Furthermore, the groups M and H do not differ significantly, as they share a common letter. These conclusions are in line with the previous results obtained in Figure 3.2.

CHAPTER 4

Applications

In this chapter we use several applications to illustrate the multiple hypotheses testing framework developed in Chapter 3 for general parametric models. The combination of the methods from Chapter 3 with the closure principle described in Section 2.2.3 leads to powerful stepwise procedures, which form the core methodology for analyzing the examples in this chapter. At the same time we illustrate the capabilities of the **multcomp** package in R, which provides an efficient implementation of these methods.

In Section 4.1 we approach the common problem of comparing several groups with a control and describe the Dunnett test. In Section 4.2 we consider the equally important problem of all pairwise comparisons for several groups and describe the Tukey test. Sections 4.1 and 4.2 both focus on important applications and accordingly we discuss the illustrating examples in detail. In addition, we describe stepwise extensions, which lead to more powerful procedures than the original Dunnett and Tukey tests. The developed methods are very general, hold for any type of comparison within the framework from Chapter 3, and are available in **multcomp**.

In the remainder of this chapter we illustrate the conduct of multiple comparison procedures for the general linear and parametric models from Chapter 3, including a number of applications beyond the common ANOVA or regression setting, as discussed in Hothorn et al. (2008). In Section 4.3 we consider an ANCOVA example of a dose response study with two covariates. Here, we focus on the evaluation of non-pairwise contrast tests as opposed to the preceeding two sections, where we were only interested in pairwise comparisons. In Section 4.4 we use a body fat prediction example to illustrate the application of multiple comparison procedures to variable selection in linear regression models. In Section 4.5 we consider the comparison of two linear regression models using simultaneous confidence bands. In Section 4.6 we look at all pairwise comparisons of expression levels for various genetic conditions of alcoholism in a heteroscedastic one-way ANOVA model using sandwich estimators. In Section 4.7 we use logistic regression to estimate the probability of suffering from Alzheimer's disease. In Section 4.8 we compare several risk factors for survival of leukemia patients using a Weibull model. Finally, in Section 4.9 we obtain probability estimates of deer browsing for various tree species from mixed-effects models.

The examples in this chapter are self-contained. Readers, who only glanced through Chapters 2 and Chapter 3, should be able to follow the examples and apply the techniques (and, in particular, the relevant function calls using

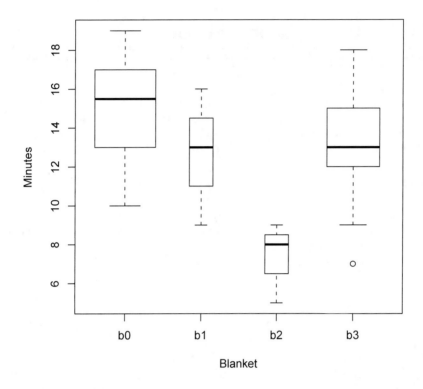

Figure 4.1   Boxplots of the `recovery` data.

multcomp) to their own problems. Theoretical results are linked back to previous chapters, where necessary. For details on the **multcomp** package we refer to Section 3.3.

4.1 Multiple comparisons with a control

In this section we consider the problem of comparing several groups with a common control group in an unbalanced one-way layout. In Section 4.1.1 we introduce the well-known Dunnett test, which is the standard method in this situation. In Section 4.1.2 we then consider a stepwise extension of the Dunnett test based on the closure principle, which is more powerful than the original Dunnett test.

4.1.1 Dunnett test

To illustrate the *Dunnett test* we consider the **recovery** data from Westfall et al. (1999). A company developed specialized heating blankets designed to help the body heat following a surgical procedure. Four types of blankets b_0, b_1, b_2, and b_3 were tested on surgical patients to assess recovery times. The blanket b_0 was a standard blanket already in use at various hospitals. The primary outcome of interest was recovery time in minutes of patients allocated randomly to one of the four treatments. Lower recovery times would indicate a better treatment effect.

The **recovery** dataset is available from the **multcomp** package,

```
R> data("recovery", package = "multcomp")
R> summary(recovery)
```

```
 blanket      minutes
 b0:20    Min.    : 5.0
 b1: 3    1st Qu.:12.0
 b2: 3    Median :13.0
 b3:15    Mean    :13.5
          3rd Qu.:16.0
          Max.    :19.0
```

As seen from the summary above, the group sample sizes differ considerably: 20 patients received blanket b_0, 3 patients received blanket b_1, another 3 patients received blanket b_2, and 15 patients received blanket b_3. Figure 4.1 displays the boxplots for the **recovery** data. We conclude from the boxplots that the observations are approximately normally distributed with equal group variances. Blanket b_2 seems to reduce the mean recovery time as compared to the standard blanket b_0, but we want to make this claim while controlling the familywise error rate with a suitable multiple comparison procedure.

To analyze the data more formally we assume the unbalanced one-way layout

$$y_{ij} = \gamma + \mu_i + \varepsilon_{ij} \qquad (4.1)$$

with independent, homoscedastic and normally distributed residual errors $\varepsilon_{ij} \sim N(0, \sigma^2)$. In Equation (4.1), y_{ij} denotes the j-th observation in treatment group i, $j = 1, \ldots, n_i$, where n_i denotes the sample size of group i, γ denotes the intercept (i.e., the overall mean), and μ_i denotes the mean effect of treatment group $i = 0, \ldots, 3$. Note that model (4.1) is a special case of the general linear model (3.1), where

$$
\mathbf{y} = \begin{pmatrix} 15 \\ 13 \\ \vdots \\ 12 \\ 13 \\ \vdots \\ 9 \\ 14 \\ \vdots \\ 13 \end{pmatrix}, \quad \mathbf{X} = \begin{pmatrix} 1 & 1 & 0 & 0 & 0 \\ 1 & 1 & 0 & 0 & 0 \\ \vdots & \vdots & \vdots & \vdots & \vdots \\ 1 & 1 & 0 & 0 & 0 \\ 1 & 0 & 1 & 0 & 0 \\ \vdots & \vdots & \vdots & \vdots & \vdots \\ 1 & 0 & 0 & 1 & 0 \\ 1 & 0 & 0 & 0 & 1 \\ \vdots & \vdots & \vdots & \vdots & \vdots \\ 1 & 0 & 0 & 0 & 1 \end{pmatrix}, \quad \text{and} \quad \boldsymbol{\beta} = \begin{pmatrix} \gamma \\ \mu_0 \\ \mu_1 \\ \mu_2 \\ \mu_3 \end{pmatrix}.
$$

The natural question of this study is whether any of the blanket types b_1, b_2, or b_3 significantly reduces the recovery time compared with b_0. This is the classical *many-to-one* problem of comparing several treatments with a control. Thus, we are interested in testing the three one-sided null hypotheses

$$
H_i: \mu_0 \leq \mu_i, \quad i = 1, 2, 3.
$$

The null hypothesis H_i therefore indicates that the mean recovery time for blanket b_0 is lower than it is for blanket b_i. Accordingly, the alternative hypotheses are given by

$$
K_i: \mu_0 > \mu_i, \quad i = 1, 2, 3.
$$

Rejecting any of the three null hypotheses H_i thus ensures that at least one of the new blankets is better than the standard b_0 at a given confidence level $1 - \alpha$, if suitable multiple comparison procedures are employed.

The standard multiple comparison procedure to address the many-to-one problem is the Dunnett (1955) test. In essence, the one-sided Dunnett test takes the minimum (or the maximum, depending on the sideness of the test problem) of the m, say, pairwise t tests

$$
t_i = \frac{\bar{y}_i - \bar{y}_0}{s\sqrt{\frac{1}{n_i} + \frac{1}{n_0}}}, \quad i = 1, \ldots, m, \tag{4.2}
$$

where $\bar{y}_i = \sum_{j=1}^{n_i} y_{ij}/n_i$ denotes the arithmetic mean of group $i = 0, \ldots, m$, and $s^2 = \sum_{i=0}^{m} \sum_{j=1}^{n_i} (y_{ij} - \bar{y}_i)^2/\nu$ denotes the pooled variance estimate with $\nu = \sum_{i=0}^{m} n_i - (m + 1)$ degrees of freedom. Note that these are the standard expressions for one-way ANOVA models, which are special cases of the more general expressions (3.3) and (3.4). In the `recovery` data example, we have $m = 3$ treatment-control comparisons, leading to three test statistics of the form (4.2).

As immediately seen from expression (4.2), each test statistic t_i is univariate t distributed. The vector of test statistics $\mathbf{t} = (t_1, \ldots, t_m)$ follows an m-variate t distribution with ν degrees of freedom and correlation matrix $\mathbf{R} = (\rho_{ij})_{ij}$, where for $i \neq j$

$$\rho_{ij} = \sqrt{\frac{n_i}{n_i + n_0}} \sqrt{\frac{n_j}{n_j + n_0}}, \quad i, j = 1, \ldots, m. \tag{4.3}$$

In the balanced case, $n_0 = n_1 = \ldots = n_m$ and the correlations are constant, $\rho_{ij} = 0.5$ for all $i \neq j$. As discussed in Chapter 3, either multidimensional integration routines, such as those from Genz and Bretz (2009), or user-friendly interfaces on top of such routines, such as the **multcomp** package in R, can be used to calculate adjusted p-values or critical values.

In the following we show how to analyze the `recovery` data with **multcomp**. We start fitting an ANOVA model by calling the `aov` function

```
R> recovery.aov <- aov(minutes ~ blanket, data = recovery)
```

The `glht` function from **multcomp** takes the fitted response model to perform the multiple comparisons through

```
R> library("multcomp")
R> recovery.mc <- glht(recovery.aov,
+                      linfct = mcp(blanket = "Dunnett"),
+                      alternative = "less")
```

In the previous call, we used the `mcp` function for the `linfct` argument to specify the comparisons type (i.e., the contrast matrix) we are interested in. The syntax is almost self-descriptive: Specify the factor of relevance (`blanket` in our example) and select one of several pre-defined contrast matrices; see the applications discussed in the subsequent sections of this chapter for other examples of pre-defined comparison types. Because we have a one-sided test problem and we are interested in showing a reduction in recovery time, we have to pass the `alternative = "less"` argument to `glht`.

We obtain a detailed summary of the results by using the `summary` method associated with the `glht` function,

```
R> summary(recovery.mc)
```

```
        Simultaneous Tests for General Linear Hypotheses

Multiple Comparisons of Means: Dunnett Contrasts


Fit: aov(formula = minutes ~ blanket, data = recovery)

Linear Hypotheses:
             Estimate Std. Error t value Pr(<t)
b1 - b0 >= 0   -2.133      1.604   -1.33   0.241
b2 - b0 >= 0   -7.467      1.604   -4.66  <0.001 ***
b3 - b0 >= 0   -1.667      0.885   -1.88   0.092 .
---
Signif. codes:  0 '***' 0.001 '**' 0.01 '*' 0.05 '.' 0.1 ' ' 1
(Adjusted p values reported -- single-step method)
```

The main part of the output consists of a table with three rows, one for each of the $m = 3$ hypotheses. From left to right we have a short descriptor of the comparisons, the effect estimates with associated standard errors and the test statistics, as defined in Equation (4.2). Multiplicity adjusted p-values are reported in the last column. By default, these p-values are calculated from the underlying multivariate t distribution (thus accounting for the correlations between the test statistics) and can be compared directly with the pre-specified significance level α. For the recovery example we conclude at level $\alpha = 0.05$ that blanket b_2 leads to significantly lower recovery times as compared with the standard blanket b_0.

For the purpose of illustration, we compare the Dunnett test with the standard Bonferroni approach. Recall that the Bonferroni approach does not account for the correlations between the test statistics (Section 2.3.1) and is thus less powerful than the Dunnett test. With the **multcomp** package we can apply the Bonferroni approach by using the `adjusted` option from the `summary` method,

```
R> summary(recovery.mc, test = adjusted(type = "bonferroni"))
```

```
        Simultaneous Tests for General Linear Hypotheses

Multiple Comparisons of Means: Dunnett Contrasts


Fit: aov(formula = minutes ~ blanket, data = recovery)

Linear Hypotheses:
             Estimate Std. Error t value  Pr(<t)
b1 - b0 >= 0   -2.133      1.604   -1.33    0.29
b2 - b0 >= 0   -7.467      1.604   -4.66 6.1e-05 ***
b3 - b0 >= 0   -1.667      0.885   -1.88    0.10
---
Signif. codes:  0 '***' 0.001 '**' 0.01 '*' 0.05 '.' 0.1 ' ' 1
(Adjusted p values reported -- bonferroni method)
```

As expected, the adjusted p-values for the Dunnett test are uniformly smaller than those from the Bonferroni adjustment. The differences in p-values are not that large in this example because of the relatively small correlations $\rho_{12} = 0.13, \rho_{13} = 0.236$, and $\rho_{23} = 0.236$; see Equation (4.3).

Next, we compute 95% one-sided simultaneous confidence intervals for the mean effect differences $\mu_i - \mu_0$, $i = 1, 2, 3$. It follows from Section 3.1.1 that for the Dunnett test these are given by

$$\left(-\infty; \; \bar{y}_i - \bar{y}_0 + u_{1-\alpha} \, s \sqrt{\frac{1}{n_i} + \frac{1}{n_0}} \, \right],$$

where $u_{1-\alpha}$ denotes the $(1 - \alpha)$-quantile from the multivariate t distribution with the correlations (4.3). Alternatively, we can use the `confint` method associated with the `glht` function,

```
R> recovery.ci <- confint(recovery.mc, level = 0.95)
R> recovery.ci
```

```
        Simultaneous Confidence Intervals

Multiple Comparisons of Means: Dunnett Contrasts


Fit: aov(formula = minutes ~ blanket, data = recovery)

Quantile = 2.18
95% family-wise confidence level


Linear Hypotheses:
             Estimate lwr      upr
b1 - b0 >= 0 -2.133      -Inf   1.367
b2 - b0 >= 0 -7.467      -Inf  -3.966
b3 - b0 >= 0 -1.667      -Inf   0.265
```

We conclude from the output that only the upper confidence bound for $\mu_2 - \mu_0$ is negative, reflecting the previous test decision that blanket b_2 leads to a significant reduction in recovery time compared with the standard blanket b_0. Moreover, we conclude at the designated confidence level of 95% that the mean recovery time for b_2 is at least 4 minutes shorter than for b_0. In addition, we can display the confidence intervals graphically with

```
R> plot(recovery.ci, main = "", ylim = c(0.5, 3.5),
+         xlab = "Minutes")
```

see Figure 4.2 for the resulting plot.

As explained in Section 3.3.1, there are several ways to specify the comparisons of interest. A convenient way is to call pre-defined contrast matrices, as done above when selecting the mcp(blanket = "Dunnett") option for the linfct argument. Alternatively, we can directly specify the contrast matrix $\mathbf{C}$ reflecting the comparisons of interest. The contrast matrix associated with the many-to-one comparisons for the levels of the factor blanket is given by

$$\mathbf{C}^\top = \begin{pmatrix} -1 & 1 & 0 & 0 \\ -1 & 0 & 1 & 0 \\ -1 & 0 & 0 & 1 \end{pmatrix},$$

such that

$$\mathbf{C}^\top \begin{pmatrix} \mu_0 \\ \mu_1 \\ \mu_2 \\ \mu_3 \end{pmatrix} = \begin{pmatrix} \mu_1 - \mu_0 \\ \mu_2 - \mu_0 \\ \mu_3 - \mu_0 \end{pmatrix}$$

leads to the pairwise comparisons of interest. Using **multcomp**, we first define the contrast matrix manually and then call the glht function,

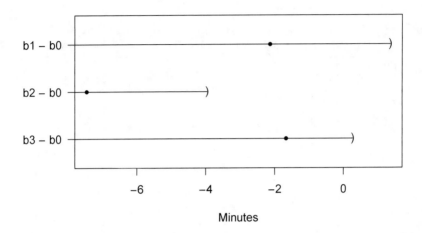

Figure 4.2   One-sided simultaneous confidence intervals for the Dunnett test in
the recovery example.

```
R> contr <- rbind("b1 -b0" = c(-1, 1, 0, 0),
+                 "b2 -b0" = c(-1, 0, 1, 0),
+                 "b3 -b0" = c(-1, 0, 0, 1))
R> summary(glht(recovery.aov, linfct = mcp(blanket = contr),
+           alternative = "less"))
```

           Simultaneous Tests for General Linear Hypotheses

Multiple Comparisons of Means: User-defined Contrasts

Fit: aov(formula = minutes ~ blanket, data = recovery)

Linear Hypotheses:
                 Estimate Std. Error t value Pr(<t)
b1 -b0 >= 0   -2.133   1.604   -1.33   0.241
*b2 -b0 >= 0   -7.467   1.604   -4.66 <0.001 ****
b3 -b0 >= 0   -1.667   0.885   -1.88   0.093 .
---
*Signif. codes: 0 '***' 0.001 '**' 0.01 '*' 0.05 '.' 0.1 ' ' 1*
(Adjusted p values reported -- single-step method)

As expected, we obtain the same adjusted p-values as in the previous call with
the mcp(blanket = "Dunnett") option for the linfct argument.

   The advantage of defining the contrast matrix manually is the retained flexibility to perform multiple comparisons which are less often applied in practice and thus not pre-defined in **multcomp**. To illustrate this advantage, consider the following modification of the `recovery` example. Suppose that both blankets b_0 and b_1 are standard treatments. Assume further that we are interested in comparing the two new blankets b_2 and b_3 with both b_0 and b_1. The original Dunnett test is not applicable, because it assumes only a single control treatment. Comparing several treatments with more than one control group was investigated by Solorzano and Spurrier (1999) and Spurrier and Solorzano (2004). With **multcomp** we can simply specify the comparison type ourselves and run the `glht` function as done above for the Dunnett test. To illustrate this, assume that we want to compare each of the new blankets b_2 and b_3 with both b_0 and b_1, resulting in a total of $m = 4$ comparisons. Accordingly,

```
R> contr2 <- rbind("b2 -b0" = c(-1,  0, 1, 0),
+                  "b2 -b1" = c( 0, -1, 1, 0),
+                  "b3 -b0" = c(-1,  0, 0, 1),
+                  "b3 -b1" = c( 0, -1, 0, 1))
```

defines the contrast matrix of interest and we pass `contr2` to `mcp`,

```
R> summary(glht(recovery.aov, linfct = mcp(blanket = contr2),
+               alternative = "less"))
```

```
        Simultaneous Tests for General Linear Hypotheses

Multiple Comparisons of Means: User-defined Contrasts


Fit: aov(formula = minutes ~ blanket, data = recovery)

Linear Hypotheses:
            Estimate Std. Error t value Pr(<t)
b2 -b0 >= 0   -7.467      1.604   -4.66 <0.001 ***
b2 -b1 >= 0   -5.333      2.115   -2.52  0.027 *
b3 -b0 >= 0   -1.667      0.885   -1.88  0.105
b3 -b1 >= 0    0.467      1.638    0.28  0.915
---
Signif. codes:  0 '***' 0.001 '**' 0.01 '*' 0.05 '.' 0.1 ' ' 1
(Adjusted p values reported -- single-step method)
```

The output gives the correct results for this multiple comparison problem and we conclude that blanket b_2 is better than both b_0 and b_1.

4.1.2 Step-down Dunnett test procedure

In Section 4.1.1 we considered the original Dunnett test, which is a single-step test. As explained in Section 2.1.2, stepwise extensions of single-step multiple comparison procedures are often available and lead to more powerful methods in the sense that they reject at least as many hypotheses as their single-step counterparts. Step-down extensions of the original Dunnett test were investigated by Naik (1975); Marcus et al. (1976); Dunnett and Tamhane (1991) and others. Step-up versions of the Dunnett test are also available (Dunnett and Tamhane 1991) but will not be considered here. In the following, we apply the closure principle described in Section 2.2.3 to the many-to-one comparison problem, give a general step-down testing algorithm based on max-t tests (which includes the Dunnett test as a special case) and then come back to the **recovery** data example to illustrate the step-down Dunnett test, which is also available in the **multcomp** package.

To make the ideas concrete, recall the $m = 3$ null hypotheses $H_i : \mu_0 \leq \mu_i$, $i = 1, 2, 3$, in the recovery example from Section 4.1.1. Following the closure principle, we construct from the set $\mathcal{H} = \{H_1, H_2, H_3\}$ of elementary null hypotheses the full closure $\bar{\mathcal{H}} = \{H_1, H_2, H_3, H_{12}, H_{13}, H_{23}, H_{123}\}$ of all intersection hypotheses $H_I = \bigcap_{i \in I} H_i, I \subseteq \{1, 2, 3\}$. The closure principle demands that we reject an elementary null hypothesis $H_i, i = 1, 2, 3$, only, if all intersection hypotheses $H_I \in \bar{\mathcal{H}}$ with $i \in I$ are rejected by their local α-level tests. For example, in order to reject H_1, we need to ensure that all intersection hypotheses contained in H_1 are also rejected (i.e., H_{12}, H_{13}, and H_{123}). This induces a natural top-down testing order; see also Figure 4.3 for a visualization of the resulting closed test procedure. We start with testing H_{123}. If we do not reject H_{123}, none of the elementary hypotheses H_1, H_2, H_3 can be rejected and the procedure stops. Otherwise, we reject H_{123} and continue testing one level down, that is, all pairwise intersection hypotheses H_{12}, H_{13}, H_{23}; and so on.

We have not mentioned before, which tests to use for the intersection hypotheses. Consider in more detail the global intersection hypothesis

$$H_{123} = H_1 \cap H_2 \cap H_3 : \mu_0 \leq \mu_1 \text{ and } \mu_0 \leq \mu_2 \text{ and } \mu_0 \leq \mu_3, \qquad (4.4)$$

which states that the blanket types b_1, b_2, and b_3 are all inferior to the standard blanket b_0. If at least one of the new blankets is superior to b_0 and reduces the recovery time, the null hypothesis H_{123} would no longer be true and we would like to reject it with high probability. This is the union intersection setting discussed in Section 2.2.1. A natural approach is to consider the minimum of the m standardized pairwise differences t_i from Equation (4.2), leading to max-t tests of the form (2.1); recall that we keep the common term "max-t" regardless of the sideness of the test problem. Thus, we can use the single-step Dunnett test (which, of course, is a max-t test) for the global intersection hypothesis H_{123}. Similarly, we can apply the Dunnett test for any of the pairwise intersection hypotheses H_{12}, H_{13}, and H_{23} while only accounting for the pair of treatment groups involved in the respective intersection. Finally, the elementary hypotheses H_1, H_2, and H_3 are tested using the t tests from Equation (4.2). This leads to a closed test procedure which uses Dunnett tests for each intersection hypothesis (adjusted for the number of treatments entering the corresponding intersection).

As mentioned in Section 2.2.1, however, a particularly appealing property of max-t tests is that they admit shortcuts of the full closure, significantly reducing the complexity. In other words, if m null hypotheses satisfying the free combination condition (which is true for many-to-one comparison problems; see Section 2.1.2) are tested with max-t tests, shortcuts of size m can be applied. This avoids testing the $2^m - 1$ intersection hypotheses in the full closure. Below we give a general step-down algorithm to test m hypotheses under the free combination condition, assuming that larger values of t_i favour the rejection of H_i. For two-sided and lower-sided test problems the $\arg\max_i t_i$ operations have to be modified accordingly.

Step-down algorithm based on max-t tests under the free combination condition

Step 1: Test the global intersection hypothesis $H_{I_1} = \bigcap_{i \in I_1} H_i$, $I_1 = \{1, \ldots, m\}$, with a suitable max-t test, resulting in the p-value p_{I_1}; if $p_{I_1} \leq \alpha$, reject H_{i_1} with adjusted p-value $q_{i_1} = p_{I_1}$ and proceed, where $i_1 = \arg\max_{i \in I_1} t_i$; otherwise stop.

Step 2: Let $I_2 = I_1 \setminus \{i_1\}$. Test $H_{I_2} = \bigcap_{i \in I_2} H_i$ with a suitable max-t test, resulting in the p-value p_{I_2}; if $p_{I_2} \leq \alpha$, reject H_{i_2} with adjusted p-value $q_{i_2} = \max\{q_{i_1}, p_{I_2}\}$ and proceed, where $i_2 = \arg\max_{i \in I_2} t_i$; otherwise stop.

$$\vdots$$

Step j: Let $I_j = I_{j-1} \setminus \{i_{j-1}\}$. Test $H_{I_j} = \bigcap_{i \in I_j} H_i$ with a suitable max-t test resulting in the p-value p_{I_j}; if $p_{I_j} \leq \alpha$, reject H_{i_j} with adjusted p-value $q_{i_j} = \max\{q_{i_{j-1}}, p_{I_j}\}$ and proceed, where $i_j = \arg\max_{i \in I_j} t_i$; otherwise stop.

$$\vdots$$

Step m: Let $I_m = I_{m-1} \setminus \{i_{m-1}\} = \{i_m\}$. Test H_{i_m} with a t test, resulting in the p-value p_{i_m}; if $p_{i_m} \leq \alpha$, reject H_{i_m} with adjusted p-value $q_{i_m} = \max\{q_{i_{m-1}}, p_{i_m}\}$; the procedure stops in any case.

The Holm procedure described in Section 2.3.2 is a well-known example of this algorithm, because it repeatedly applies Bonferroni's inequality in at most m steps (recall that the Bonferroni method is also a max-t test). However, because the Bonnferroni method does not account for the correlations between the test statistics, the Holm procedure can be improved. By applying Dunnett tests at each step for the many-to-one comparison problem of the `recovery` example, we obtain the powerful *step-down Dunnett procedure*.

To illustrate the step-down Dunnett test, consider Figure 4.3, which shows the closed representation of the Dunnett tests for the `recovery` example. The observed one-sided t statistics shown at the bottom level for the comparisons with the control are $t_1^{\text{obs}} = -1.33$, $t_2^{\text{obs}} = -4.656$, and $t_3^{\text{obs}} = -1.884$, respectively for the `b1` - `b0`, `b2` - `b0`, and `b3` - `b0` comparisons. At the top level, the global intersection hypothesis (4.4) is H_{I_1} in *Step 1* of the step-down algorithm, where $I_1 = \{1, 2, 3\}$. We test H_{123} using $t_{123}^{\text{obs}} = -4.656$, which is highly significant with $p_{123} = \mathbb{P}(\min\{t_1, t_2, t_3\} \leq -4.656) < 0.001$. This allows one to use a shortcut for the rest of the tree for tests that include the `b2` - `b0` comparison: It follows from $\mathbb{P}(\min\{t_1, t_2, t_3\} \leq -4.656) < 0.001$ that $\mathbb{P}(\min\{t_1, t_2\} \leq -4.656) < 0.001$, $\mathbb{P}(\min\{t_2, t_3\} \leq -4.656) < 0.001$, and $\mathbb{P}(t_2 \leq -4.656) < 0.001$. Hence, all intersection hypotheses including the `b2` - `b0` comparison can be rejected by virtue of rejecting the global null hypothesis. Thus, the `b2` - `b0` comparison can itself be deemed significant. This logic explains *Step 1* of the step-down algorithm above. The remaining steps are explained similarly. In the notation from the step-down algorithm, $i_1 = 2$ and consequently $I_2 = I_1 \setminus \{2\} = \{1, 3\}$. Consider Figure 4.3 again. The remaining non-rejected pairwise intersection hypothesis is H_{13}: $\mu_0 \leq \mu_1$ and $\mu_0 \leq \mu_3$. The related test statistic is $t_{13}^{\text{obs}} = -1.884$ with $p_{13} = \mathbb{P}(\min\{t_1, t_3\} \leq -1.884) = 0.064$. Thus, we cannot reject H_{13} at significance level $\alpha = 0.05$, which renders further testing unnecessary. This logic explains *Step 2* of the algorithm, and, because we cannot reject at this step, we have to terminate the step-down procedure.

In summary, we conclude from this example that step-down procedures are special cases of closed test procedures and that the use of max-t tests allows for shortcuts to the full closure, where only the subsets corresponding to the ordered test statistics need to be tested. Note that the step-down algorithm presented here is valid under the free combination condition; for restricted hypotheses we refer to the discussion in Section 4.2.2.

We conclude this section by showing how to invoke the step-down Dunnett test with the **multcomp** package using the `recovery` data. The step-down algorithm for hypotheses satisfying the free combination condition is available with the `adjusted(type = "free")` option in the `summary` method

```
R> summary(recovery.mc, test = adjusted(type = "free"))
```

```
        Simultaneous Tests for General Linear Hypotheses

Multiple Comparisons of Means: Dunnett Contrasts


Fit: aov(formula = minutes ~ blanket, data = recovery)

Linear Hypotheses:
             Estimate Std. Error t value Pr(<t)
b1 - b0 >= 0   -2.133      1.604   -1.33  0.096 .
b2 - b0 >= 0   -7.467      1.604   -4.66  6e-05 ***
b3 - b0 >= 0   -1.667      0.885   -1.88  0.064 .
---
```

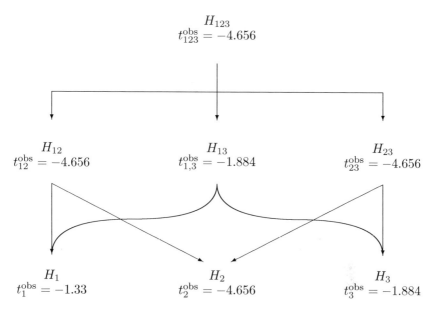

Figure 4.3   Closed Dunnett test in the **recovery** example.

```
Signif. codes:   0 '***' 0.001 '**' 0.01 '*' 0.05 '.' 0.1 ' ' 1
(Adjusted p values reported -- free method)
```

The results from the output above match the results from the previous discussion. In particular, the step-down Dunnett test provides substantially smaller adjusted p-values than the single-step Dunnett test from Section 4.1.1; see also Table 4.1 for a side-by-side comparison. In Table 4.1 we have also included for illustration purposes the unadjusted p-values p_i as well as the adjusted p-values from the Bonferroni test and the Holm procedure

```
R> summary(recovery.mc, test = adjusted(type = "holm"))
```

Both step-down procedures (Holm, step-down Dunnett) are clearly more powerful than their single-step counterparts (Bonferroni, Dunnett). In addition, we conclude from Table 4.1 that methods accounting for correlations between the test statistics (Dunnett, step-down Dunnett) are more powerful than methods which do not (Bonferroni, Holm). As explained in Section 4.1.1, the correlations are fairly small in this example and thus the Bonferroni-based procedures behave reasonably well. Finally, note that simultaneous confidence intervals for stepwise procedures are not implemented in **multcomp**, since they are typically hard to compute, if available at all. Simultaneous confidence intervals have been investigated by Bofinger (1987) for the step-down Dunnett procedure and by Strassburger and Bretz (2008) and Guilbaud (2008) for the Holm procedure.

Comparison	p_i	Adjusted p-values q_i			
		Bonferroni	Dunnett	Holm	step-down Dunnett
b1 - b0	0.096	0.287	0.241	0.096	0.096
b2 - b0	0.001	0.001	0.001	0.001	0.001
b3 - b0	0.034	0.101	0.092	0.067	0.064

Table 4.1   Comparison of several multiple comparison procedures for the `recovery` data.

4.2 All pairwise comparisons

In this section we consider all pairwise comparisons of several means in a two-way layout. In Section 4.2.1 we introduce the well-known Tukey test, which is the standard procedure in this situation. In Section 4.2.2 we consider a stepwise extension based on the closure principle, which is more powerful than the original Tukey test.

4.2.1 Tukey test

To illustrate the *Tukey test* we consider the `immer` data from Venables and Ripley (2002) describing a field experiment on barley yields. Five varieties of barley were grown in six locations in both 1931 and 1932. Following Venables and Ripley (2002), we average the results for the two years. To analyze the data we consider the two-way layout

$$y_{ij} = \gamma + \mu_i + \alpha_j + \varepsilon_{ij} \tag{4.5}$$

with independent, homoscedastic and normally distributed residual errors $\varepsilon_{ij} \sim N(0, \sigma^2)$. In Equation (4.5), y_{ij} denotes the average barley yield for variety i at location j, γ the intercept (i.e., the overall mean), μ_i the mean effect of variety $i = 1, \ldots, 5$, and α_j the mean effect of location $j = 1, \ldots, 6$. Note that model (4.5) is a special case of the general linear model (3.1), where

$$
\mathbf{y} = \begin{pmatrix} 109.35 \\ 77.30 \\ \vdots \\ 123.50 \\ 100.25 \\ \vdots \\ 131.45 \end{pmatrix}, \quad
\mathbf{X} = \begin{pmatrix}
1 & 1 & 0 & \ldots & 0 & 1 & 0 & \ldots & 0 \\
1 & 1 & 0 & \ldots & 0 & 0 & 1 & \ldots & 0 \\
\vdots & \vdots & \vdots & \ldots & \vdots & \vdots & \vdots & \ldots & \vdots \\
1 & 1 & 0 & \ldots & 0 & 0 & 0 & \ldots & 1 \\
1 & 0 & 1 & \ldots & 0 & 1 & 0 & \ldots & 0 \\
\vdots & \vdots & \vdots & \ldots & \vdots & \vdots & \vdots & \ldots & \vdots \\
1 & 0 & 0 & \ldots & 1 & 0 & 0 & \ldots & 1
\end{pmatrix},
$$

and $\boldsymbol{\beta} = (\gamma, \mu_1, \ldots, \mu_5, \alpha_1, \ldots, \alpha_6)^\top$.

The `immer` data are available with the **MASS** package (Venables and Ripley 2002). Consequently, we can run a standard analysis of variance using the `aov` function as follows:

```
R> data("immer", package = "MASS")
R> immer.aov <- aov((Y1 + Y2)/2 ~ Var + Loc, data = immer)
R> summary(immer.aov)
            Df Sum Sq Mean Sq F value  Pr(>F)
Var          4   2655     664    5.99  0.0025 **
Loc          5  10610    2122   19.15 5.2e-07 ***
Residuals   20   2217     111
---
Signif. codes:  0 '***' 0.001 '**' 0.01 '*' 0.05 '.' 0.1 ' ' 1
```

The ANOVA F tests indicate that both Var and Loc have a significant effect on the average barley yield. Following Venables and Ripley (2002), we are interested in comparing the $k = 5$ varieties with each other while averaging the results for the two years, resulting in $k(k-1)/2 = 10$ pairwise comparisons. We can retrieve the mean yields for the five varieties by a call to model.tables

```
R> model.tables(immer.aov, type = "means")$tables$Var
Var
    M     P     S     T     V
 94.4 102.5  91.1 118.2  99.2
```

This leads to the classical *all-pairwise comparison* problem. We are thus interested in testing the 10 two-sided null hypotheses

$$H_{ij}\colon \mu_i = \mu_j, \quad i,j \in \{M,P,S,T,V\}, i \neq j.$$

The null hypothesis H_{ij} indicates that the mean yield in barley does not differ for the varieties i and j. Accordingly, the alternative hypotheses are given by

$$K_{ij}\colon \mu_i \neq \mu_j, \quad i,j \in \{M,P,S,T,V\}, i \neq j.$$

Rejecting any of the 10 null hypotheses H_{ij} ensures that at least two of the five varieties differ with respect to their average yield. We make this claim at a given confidence level $1 - \alpha$, if we employ suitable multiple comparison procedures. The standard multiple comparison procedure to address the all-pairwise comparison problem is the Tukey (1953) test, also known as *studentized range test*. Note that some textbooks suggest performing the Tukey test only after observing a significant ANOVA F test result. We recommend using the methods described below, regardless of whether or not the ANOVA F test is significant.

In essence, the Tukey test takes the maximum over the absolute values of all pairwise test statistics, which in the completely randomized layout of the immer example take the form

$$t_{ij} = \frac{\bar{y}_i - \bar{y}_j}{s\sqrt{\frac{2}{n}}}. \tag{4.6}$$

In the last expression, $\bar{y}_i$ denotes the least squares mean estimate for variety i (which coincides with the usual arithmetic mean estimate in this case), s the pooled standard deviation and n the common sample size, that is, $n = 6$ as we have six locations and one observation for each combination of variety and location; see Equations (3.3) and (3.4) for the more general expressions.

Each test statistic t_{ij} is univariate t distributed. The vector of the test statistics follows a multivariate t distribution. Until the emergence of modern computing facilities, the exact calculation of critical values for the Tukey test was only possible for limited cases. One example is the balanced independent one-way layout. Hayter (1984) proved analytically that in cases, where the covariance matrix of the mean estimates is diagonal (which includes the un-balanced one-way layout), using the critical values from the balanced case is conservative. In fact, it has been conjectured that using the balanced critical points will always be conservative. This was proved when $k = 3$ (Brown 1984) and in a more general context by Hayter (1989). However, efficient numerical integration methods, such as those from Bretz, Hayter, and Genz (2001) and Genz and Bretz (2009), or user-friendly interfaces on top of such routines, such as the **multcomp** package in R, can be used to calculate adjusted p-values or critical values without restrictions.

In the following we show how to analyze the immer data with **multcomp**. For details on the **multcomp** package we refer to Section 3.3. We use the fitted ANOVA model immer.aov and apply the glht function to perform the multiple comparisons through

```
R> immer.mc <- glht(immer.aov, linfct = mcp(Var = "Tukey"))
```

In the previous call, we used the mcp function for the linfct argument to specify the comparison type (i.e., the contrast matrix) that we are interested in. The syntax is almost self-descriptive: Specify the factor of relevance and select one of several pre-defined contrast matrices (Var = "Tukey" in our example).

We obtain a detailed summary of the results by using the summary method associated with the glht function,

```
R> summary(immer.mc)
```

```
        Simultaneous Tests for General Linear Hypotheses

Multiple Comparisons of Means: Tukey Contrasts


Fit: aov(formula = (Y1 + Y2)/2 ~ Var + Loc, data = immer)

Linear Hypotheses:
           Estimate Std. Error t value Pr(>|t|)
P - M == 0     8.15       6.08    1.34   0.6701
S - M == 0    -3.26       6.08   -0.54   0.9824
T - M == 0    23.81       6.08    3.92   0.0067 **
V - M == 0     4.79       6.08    0.79   0.9310
S - P == 0   -11.41       6.08   -1.88   0.3607
T - P == 0    15.66       6.08    2.58   0.1132
V - P == 0    -3.36       6.08   -0.55   0.9803
```

```
T - S == 0     27.07      6.08     4.45    0.0020 **
V - S == 0      8.05      6.08     1.32    0.6798
V - T == 0    -19.02      6.08    -3.13    0.0377 *
---
Signif. codes:  0 '***' 0.001 '**' 0.01 '*' 0.05 '.' 0.1 ' ' 1
(Adjusted p values reported -- single-step method)
```

The main part of the output consists of a table with 10 rows, one for each pairwise comparison. From left to right we have a short descriptor of the comparisons, the effect estimates with associated standard errors and the test statistics, as defined in Equation (4.6). Multiplicity adjusted p-values are reported in the last column. By default, these p-values are calculated from the underlying multivariate t distribution (thus accounting for the correlations between the test statistics) and can be compared directly with the pre-specified significance level α. For the immer example we conclude at level $\alpha = 0.05$ that the pairwise comparisons T - M, T - S, and V - T are all significantly different.

As an aside, we point out that the immer example can also be analyzed using the TukeyHSD function from the **stats** package. Calling

```
R> immer.mc2 <-TukeyHSD(immer.aov, which = "Var")
R> immer.mc2$Var
```

```
        diff     lwr     upr    p adj
P-M     8.15 -10.04 26.338 0.67006
S-M    -3.26 -21.45 14.929 0.98242
T-M    23.81   5.62 41.996 0.00678
V-M     4.79 -13.40 22.979 0.93102
S-P   -11.41 -29.60  6.779 0.36068
T-P    15.66  -2.53 33.846 0.11322
V-P    -3.36 -21.55 14.829 0.98035
T-S    27.07   8.88 45.254 0.00203
V-S     8.05 -10.14 26.238 0.67982
V-T   -19.02 -37.20 -0.829 0.03771
```

we conclude that the results obtained with glht are the same as those from TukeyHSD. Note however that the TukeyHSD function is specifically designed to perform the Tukey test for models with one-way structures (Hsu 1996, Section 7.1). Consequently, the TukeyHSD function lacks the flexibility of the **multcomp** package, which allows one to perform the Tukey test (and other types of contrast tests) for the general parametric models described in Chapter 3. For example, the previous call to glht can easily be changed to

```
R> glht(immer.aov, linfct = mcp(Var = "Tukey"),
+        alternative = "greater")
```

in order to perform the one-sided studentized range test investigated by Hayter (1990), which is a one-sided version of the Tukey test with potential application to dose response analyses.

We now consider the computation of 95% two-sided simultaneous confidence intervals for the mean effect differences $\mu_i - \mu_j$. It follows from Equation (4.6) that in the completely randomized layout of the `immer` example the simultaneous confidence intervals for the Tukey test are given by

$$\left[\bar{y}_i - \bar{y}_j - u_{1-\alpha}\, s\sqrt{\frac{2}{n}};\ \bar{y}_i - \bar{y}_j + u_{1-\alpha}\, s\sqrt{\frac{2}{n}} \right],$$

where $u_{1-\alpha}$ denotes the $(1 - \alpha)$-quantile of the multivariate t distribution. Alternatively, we can use the `confint` method associated with the `glht` function,

```
R> immer.ci <- confint(immer.mc, level = 0.95)
R> immer.ci
```

```
          Simultaneous Confidence Intervals

Multiple Comparisons of Means: Tukey Contrasts


Fit: aov(formula = (Y1 + Y2)/2 ~ Var + Loc, data = immer)

Quantile = 2.99
95% family-wise confidence level


Linear Hypotheses:
            Estimate  lwr       upr
P - M == 0    8.150   -10.038   26.338
S - M == 0   -3.258   -21.446   14.930
T - M == 0   23.808     5.620   41.996
V - M == 0    4.792   -13.396   22.980
S - P == 0  -11.408   -29.596    6.780
T - P == 0   15.658    -2.530   33.846
V - P == 0   -3.358   -21.546   14.830
T - S == 0   27.067     8.879   45.255
V - S == 0    8.050   -10.138   26.238
V - T == 0  -19.017   -37.205   -0.829
```

We conclude from the output that only the confidence intervals for the T - M, T - S, and V - T comparisons exclude 0, which is consistent with the previously established test results. Moreover, we conclude at the designated confidence level of 95% that the average barley yield for variety T is larger than the yield for the varieties M, S, and V. The critical value is $u_{0.95} = 2.993$. In addition, we can display the confidence intervals graphically with

```
R> plot(immer.ci, main = "", xlab = "Yield")
```

see Figure 4.4 for the resulting plot. The `plot.matchMMC` method from the **HH** package orders the confidence intervals in a different, often more intuitive way and can be used alternatively; see the bottom plot of Figure 4.7.

If the number k of treatments or conditions is large, the number of pairwise

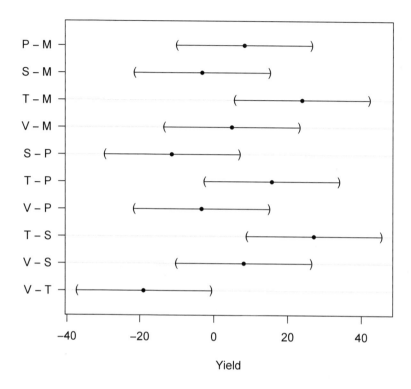

Figure 4.4 Two-sided simultaneous confidence intervals for the Tukey test in the `immer` example.

comparisons, $k(k-1)/2$, increases rapidly. In such cases, plotting the result-ing set of simultaneous confidence intervals or adjusted p-values might be too extensive and more efficient methods to display the treatment effects together with the associated significances are required. Compact letter displays are a convenient tool to provide the necessary summary information about the obtained significances. With this display, treatments are asigned letters to in-dicate significant differences. Treatments that are not significantly different are assigned a common letter. In other words, two treatments without a com-mon letter are statistically significant at the chosen significance level. Using such a letter display, an efficient presentation of the test results is available, which is often easier to communicate than extensive tables and confidence interval plots, such as those presented in Figure 4.4. Piepho (2004) provided an efficient algorithm for a compact letter-based representation of all pair-wise comparisons, which is also implemented in the **multcomp** package. This method works for general lists of pairwise p-values, regardless of how they were obtained. In particular, this method is applicable to the case of unbalanced data.

The `cld` function extracts the necessary information from `glht` objects that is required to create a compact letter display of all pairwise comparisons. Using the `immer` example from above, we can call

```
R> immer.cld <- cld(immer.mc)
```

Next, we can use the `plot` method associated with `cld` objects. Figure 4.5 shows the boxplots for each of the five varieties together with the letter display when calling

```
R> plot(immer.cld)
```

Because variety T has no letter in common with any other variety than P, it differs significantly from M, S, and V, but not from P at the chosen significance level ($\alpha = 0.05$ by default). No further significant differences can be declared, because the remaining four varieties all share the common letter b. These conclusions are in line with the previous results obtained in Figure 4.4. More details about the `cld` function are given in Section 3.3.3.

One advantage of using R is the retained flexibility to fine tune standard output. For example, one may wish to improve Figure 4.5 by ordering the boxplots according to the mean yields for the five varieties. Such ordering may enhance the readability, as treatments with common letters are more likely to be displayed side-by-side. One way of doing this is shown below; see Figure 4.6 for the resulting boxplots.

```
R> data("immer", package = "MASS")
R> library("HH")
R> immer2 <- immer
R> immer2$Var <- ordered(immer2$Var,
+     levels = c("S", "M", "V", "P", "T"))
R> immer2.aov <- aov((Y1 + Y2)/2 ~ Var + Loc, data = immer2)
R> position(immer2$Var) <- model.tables(immer2.aov,
+     type = "means")$tables$Var
R> immer2.mc  <- glht(immer2.aov, linfct = mcp(Var = "Tukey"))
R> immer2.cld <- cld(immer2.mc)
R> immer2.cld$pos.x  <- immer2.cld$x
R> position(immer2.cld$pos.x) <- position(immer2$Var)
R> lab <-
+     immer2.cld$mcletters$monospacedLetters[levels(immer2$Var)]
R> bwplot(lp ~ pos.x, data = immer2.cld,
+          panel=function(...){
+            panel.bwplot.intermediate.hh(...)
+            cpl <- current.panel.limits()
+            pushViewport(viewport(xscale = cpl$xlim,
+                                  yscale = cpl$ylim,
```

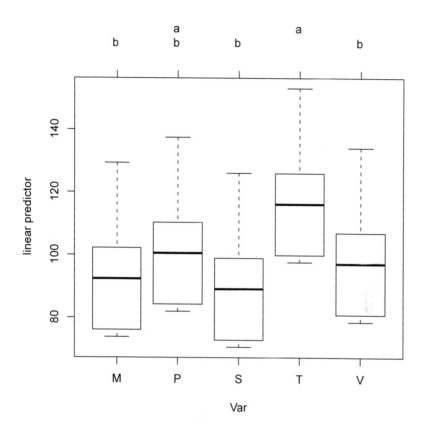

Figure 4.5 Compact letter display for all pairwise comparisons in the `immer` example.

```
+                                    clip = "off"))
+            panel.axis("top", at = position(immer2$Var),
+                     labels = lab, outside = TRUE)
+            upViewport()
+          },
+          scales = list(x = list(limits = c(90, 120),
+                     at = position(immer2$Var),
+                     labels = levels(immer2$Var))),
+       main = "", xlab = "Var", ylab = "linear predictor")
```

An alternative graphical representation of the Tukey test was developed by Hsu and Peruggia (1994) and extended to arbitrary contrasts by Heiberger and Holland (2004, 2006). The resulting mean-mean multiple comparison plot allows the display of multiple relevant information in the same plot, including

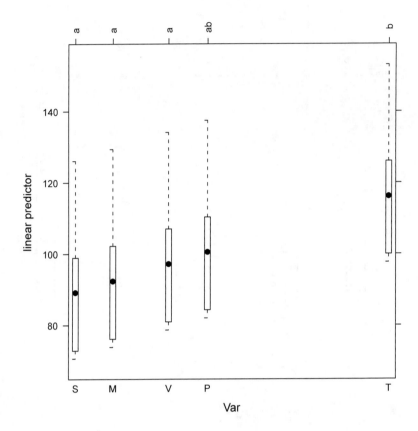

Figure 4.6   Alternative compact letter display for all pairwise comparisons in the
immer example.

the observed group mean values, with correct relative distances, and point
estimates for arbitrary contrasts together with their associated simultaneous
confidence intervals. In the following we illustrate the mean-mean multiple
comparison plot with the immer data.

Mean-mean multiple comparison plots are available with the **HH** package
(Heiberger 2009) via the glht.mmc function. Its syntax is very similar to the
one used for glht,

```
R> library("HH")
R> immer.mmc <- glht.mmc(immer.aov, linfct = mcp(Var = "Tukey"),
+                        focus = "Var", lmat.rows = 2:5)
```

In the previous statement, the focus argument defines the factor whose contrasts are to be computed. In addition, the lmat.rows argument specifies the
rows in lmat for the focus factor, where by convention lmat is the transpose

of the `linfct` component produced by `glht` (see Section 3.3.1 for details on `glht` objects). In our example,

```
R> t(immer.mc$linfct)
```

	P-M	S-M	T-M	V-M	S-P	T-P	V-P	T-S	V-S	V-T
(Intercept)	0	0	0	0	0	0	0	0	0	0
VarP	1	0	0	0	-1	-1	-1	0	0	0
VarS	0	1	0	0	1	0	0	-1	-1	0
VarT	0	0	1	0	0	1	0	1	0	-1
VarV	0	0	0	1	0	0	1	0	1	1
LocD	0	0	0	0	0	0	0	0	0	0
LocGR	0	0	0	0	0	0	0	0	0	0
LocM	0	0	0	0	0	0	0	0	0	0
LocUF	0	0	0	0	0	0	0	0	0	0
LocW	0	0	0	0	0	0	0	0	0	0

```
attr(,"type")
[1] "Tukey"
```

and we see that the Tukey contrasts for the `focus` factor `Var` are specified in rows 2 through 5; thus the `lmat.rows=2:5` specification in the `glht.mmc` call above.

With these preparations, we can display the mean-mean multiple comparison plot for the the `immer` data using

```
R> plot(immer.mmc, ry = c(85, 122), x.offset = 8,
+        main = "", main2 = "")
```

where `ry` and `x.offset` are arguments to fine tune the appearance of the plot; see the top graph in Figure 4.7 for the results. The 95% confidence intervals on $\mu_T - \mu_M$, $\mu_T - \mu_S$, and $\mu_T - \mu_V$ lie entirely to the right of 0, while all other confidence intervals include 0. We thus conclude at the 5% level that the average barley yield for variety T is larger than the yield for the varieties M, S, and V. No further significances between the varieties are uncovered, which reflects the test decisions obtained from Figure 4.4.

Each of the simultaneous confidence intervals for the 10 pairwise differences $\mu_i - \mu_j$ in Figure 4.7 is centered at a point whose height on the left y-axis is equal to the average of the corresponding means $\bar{y}_i$ and $\bar{y}_j$ and whose location along the x-axis is at distance $\bar{y}_i - \bar{y}_j$ from the vertical line at 0. Note that the confidence intervals on $\mu_P - \mu_S$ amd $\mu_V - \mu_M$ appear almost at the same height in Figure 4.7, leading to an informative overprinting of the contrast names at the right y-axis. In cases of overprinting, Heiberger and Holland (2006) suggested a tiebreaker plot of the simultaneous confidence intervals similar to Figure 4.4, where the contrasts are evenly spaced vertically in the same order as in the mean-mean multiple comparison plot and on the same horizontal scale. The tiebreaker plot for the `immer` data displayed at the bottom of Figure 4.7 was obtained with the command

```
R> plot.matchMMC(immer.mmc$mca, main = "")
```

The isomeans grid in the center of Figure 4.7 is particularly useful when

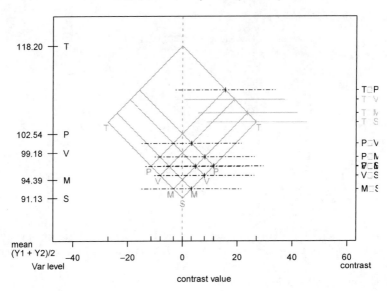

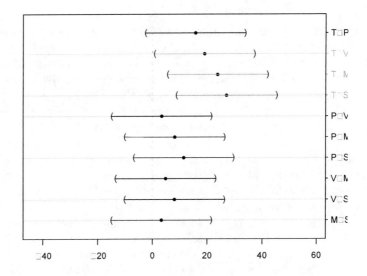

Figure 4.7   Mean-mean multiple comparison plot (top) and tiebreaker plot (bottom) for all pairwise comparisons in the `immer` example.

plotting simultaneous confidence intervals for orthogonal or more general contrasts, as shown now. It is well known that the use of carefully selected orthogonal contrasts is often preferable to a redundant set of contrasts. Because we have a total of five varieties, we can choose a basis of four orthogonal contrasts, such that any other contrast can be constructed as a linear combination of the elements of this basis set. Assume that we are interested in the four orthogonal contrasts

```
R> immer.lmat <- cbind("M-S"   = c(1, 0,-1, 0, 0),
+                      "MS-V"   = c(1, 0, 1, 0,-2),
+                      "VMS-P"  = c(1,-3, 1, 0, 1),
+                      "PVMS-T" = c(1, 1, 1,-4, 1))
R> row.names(immer.lmat) <- c("M","P","S","T","V")
```

We would like to repeat a similar analysis based on a mean-mean multiple comparison plot as done above for the Tukey test. The statement

```
R> immer.mmc2 <- glht.mmc(immer.aov, linfct = mcp(Var = "Tukey"),
+                         focus.lmat = immer.lmat)
```

is sufficient to construct the plot in Figure 4.8. Clearly, the T–PVMS comparison is highly significant, thus underpinning the previously observed good result of variety T. By comparing Figures 4.7 and 4.8, one notices that the point estimates associated with the pairwise contrasts are constructed as a linear combination of point estimates of the orthogonal contrasts. Note also that the confidence intervals in Figure 4.7 are not necessarily centered anymore at the intersections of the isomeans grid. Finally, we note that intervals obtained with the glht.mmc statement above are by default based on the conservative generalized Tukey test, which allows for selection of contrasts based on findings suggested by the pairwise analysis (Hochberg and Tamhane 1987, p. 80).

As mentioned previously, the mean-mean multiple comparison plots implemented in the **HH** package are applicable to general contrasts in factorial designs. We refer to Heiberger and Holland (2004, 2006) for further details and examples.

4.2.2 Closed Tukey test procedure

In Section 4.2.1 we considered the original Tukey test, which is a single-step test. Similar to the Dunnett test described in Section 4.1, stepwise extensions are also available for the Tukey test, leading to more power; see, for example, Finner (1988). As explained in Section 2.1.2, stepwise test procedures reject at least as many hypotheses as their single-step counterparts. In the following, we apply the closure principle described in Section 2.2.3 to the all-pairwise comparison problem, discuss efficient methods to prune the full closure and then come back to the immer data example to illustrate the closed Tukey test, which is also available in the **multcomp** package.

Recall from Section 2.2.3 that the closure principle constructs all possible intersection hypotheses from an initial set of elementary hypotheses. In some

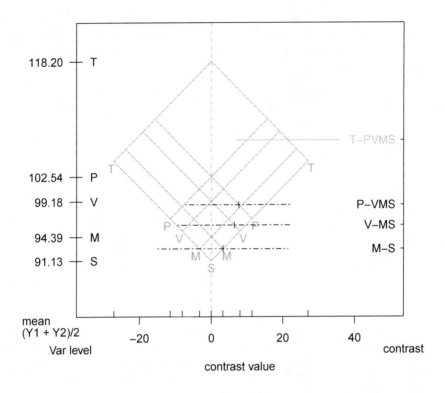

Figure 4.8 Mean-mean multiple comparison plot for selected orthogonal contrasts in the `immer` example.

cases, depending upon the structure of the hypotheses tested, the closure tree can be pruned considerably, resulting in much smaller adjusted p-values and hence more powerful tests. For example, consider the pairwise comparisons case with three groups: The basic hypotheses are $H_{12}: \mu_1 = \mu_2$, $H_{13}: \mu_1 = \mu_3$, and $H_{23}: \mu_2 = \mu_3$. As seen in Figure 2.6, these are the three elementary hypotheses. However, unlike the many-to-one case displayed in Figure 4.3, there is only one possible intersection hypothesis, rather than four, because every intersection hypothesis has the form $H_{123}: \mu_1 = \mu_2 = \mu_3$. Having fewer intersections to test implies greater power. In this case, the adjusted p-values for each of the three elementary hypotheses H_{ij} are the maximum of just two p-values: The unadjusted p-value from H_{ij} and the p-value from the global intersection hypothesis H_{123}; see Equation (2.2) for a general definition of adjusted p-values using the closure principle.

Pruning of the closure set happens when $H_I = H_{I'}$ for distinct subsets I

and I', and in this case the hypotheses are said to be restricted; see also Section 2.1.2. On the other hand, if $H_I \neq H_{I'}$ for each pair of distinct subsets I and I', then the hypotheses are said to satisfy the free combination condition. Examples of free combinations include the many-to-one comparisons considered in Section 4.1 as well as comparisons of means with two-sample multivariate data (as discussed, for example, in Section 5.1). Examples of restricted combinations include all-pairwise comparisons, response surface comparisons, and general complex contrast sets.

Figure 4.9 shows how the pruned tree looks in the case of all pairwise comparisons among four groups. The size of the tree is considerably smaller than the $2^6 - 1 = 63$ intersection hypotheses that would apply if the tests were in free combinations. Because in the restricted combination case many of the intersections produce identical intersection hypotheses, there are only 14 distinct subsets in the closure.

Shaffer (1986) presented a method for using the pruned closure tree in the case of restricted combinations to produce more powerful tests, using Bonferroni tests for each node; see also Section 2.3.2. Bergmann and Hommel (1988) extended the consept of the Shaffer procedure and found an algorithm for pruning the closure test, which was subsequently implemented by Bernhard (1992), see also Hommel and Bernhard (1992). Royen (1991) noted that the Shaffer method is in fact a *truncated closed test procedure*, where the individual tests are performed in the order of the unadjusted p-values, stopping as soon as an insignificance occurs. Hommel and Bernhard (1999) investigated more powerful closed test procedures that are obtained if testing is done without truncation, but the resulting inference may no longer be monotone in the p-values. Hommel and Bretz (2008) gave an example where a non-monotonic decision pattern still leads to a meaningful interpretation. Finally, Westfall (1997) and Westfall and Tobias (2007) showed how to perform the truncated closed test procedure for general contrasts. The method of Westfall (1997) is available in the **multcomp** package and will be illustrated below with the immer data example.

Recall from Section 4.1.2 that the step-down Dunnett procedure may be obtained as follows: (i) order the unadjusted p-values $p_{(1)} \leq \ldots \leq p_{(m)}$ as usual, corresponding to hypotheses $H_{(1)}, \ldots, H_{(m)}$; (ii) test $H_{(1)}, \ldots, H_{(m)}$ sequentially and obtain the adjusted p-values $q_{(i)} = \max_{I:i \in I} p_I$, stopping as soon as $q_{(i)} > \alpha$, where α is the desired significance level to control the familywise error rate. Truncated closed test procedures use the same method, but apply it to restricted combinations, where the set of subsets I considered in the computation of $q_{(i)} = \max_{I:i \in I} p_I$ is often much smaller than the same set under the free combination condition, leading to smaller adjusted p-values $q_{(i)}$ and hence more powerful tests. The method is called "truncated" because it is applied in the order of the adjusted p-values; it is possible to make the method even more powerful by removing this constraint. On the other hand, truncation ensures that the order of the adjusted p-values is the same as the

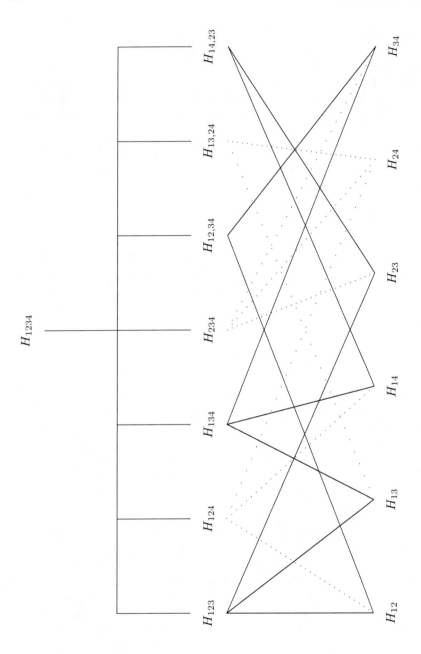

Figure 4.9   Closure principle for all pairwise comparisons of four means (schematic
diagram). Here, $H_{1234}\colon \mu_1 = \mu_2 = \mu_3 = \mu_4$, $H_{ijk}\colon \mu_i = \mu_j = \mu_k$,
$H_{\{ij\},\{k,\ell\}}\colon \mu_i = \mu_j$ and $\mu_k = \mu_\ell$, and $H_{ij}\colon \mu_i = \mu_j$ for suitable in-
dices i, j, k, and ℓ. Different line types are used to distinguish the in-
dividual implications between hypotheses and have no other meaning.

order of the unadjusated p-values; without truncation the orders may differ, leading to possible interpretation difficulties.

To illustrate the method, consider the `immer` data from above together with model (4.5). Of interest are the 10 elementary hypotheses $H_{ij}: \mu_i = \mu_j$, $i, j \in \{M, P, S, T, V\}, i \neq j$. As with the step-down Dunnett procedure, it is helpful here to express the procedure in terms of t statistics rather than p-values. Let t_{ij}^{obs} denote the observed t statistics for testing H_{ij} and let t_{ij} denote the random counterparts from Equation (4.6). For the `immer` data, the observed absolute t statistics are given in order as $t_{\mathrm{ST}}^{\mathrm{obs}} = 4.453$, $t_{\mathrm{MT}}^{\mathrm{obs}} = 3.917$, $t_{\mathrm{TV}}^{\mathrm{obs}} = 3.129$, $t_{\mathrm{PT}}^{\mathrm{obs}} = 2.576$, $t_{\mathrm{PS}}^{\mathrm{obs}} = 1.877$, $t_{\mathrm{MP}}^{\mathrm{obs}} = 1.341$, $t_{\mathrm{SV}}^{\mathrm{obs}} = 1.324$, $t_{\mathrm{MV}}^{\mathrm{obs}} = 0.788$, $t_{\mathrm{PV}}^{\mathrm{obs}} = 0.553$, $t_{\mathrm{MS}}^{\mathrm{obs}} = 0.536$. These values can be obtained from, for example, the `summary` output of the `immer.mc` object, as described in Section 4.2.1.

Using the truncated closed test procedure, we step through the related sequence of hypotheses $H_{\mathrm{ST}}, H_{\mathrm{MT}}, \ldots, H_{\mathrm{MS}}$ and test relevant subsets from the full closure using max-t tests of the form (2.1) while incorporating the parametric model results from Chapter 3. Applied to the `immer` example, we obtain the following individual steps:

(i) All subsets are strictly smaller than the global intersection set. Test H_{ST} using
$$q_{(1)} = \mathbb{P}(\max_{ij} t_{ij} \geq 4.453) = 0.002.$$

(ii) Relevant subsets and their p-values are given by
$$\mathbb{P}(\max\{t_{\mathrm{MT}}, t_{\mathrm{TV}}, t_{\mathrm{PT}}, t_{\mathrm{MP}}, t_{\mathrm{MV}}, t_{\mathrm{PV}}\} \geq 3.917) = 0.004,$$
$$\mathbb{P}(\max\{t_{\mathrm{MT}}, t_{\mathrm{PT}}, t_{\mathrm{MP}}, t_{\mathrm{SV}}\} \geq 3.917) = 0.003,$$
$$\mathbb{P}(\max\{t_{\mathrm{MT}}, t_{\mathrm{TV}}, t_{\mathrm{PS}}, t_{\mathrm{MV}}\} \geq 3.917) = 0.003, \text{ and}$$
$$\mathbb{P}(\max\{t_{\mathrm{MT}}, t_{\mathrm{PS}}, t_{\mathrm{SV}}, t_{\mathrm{PV}}\} \geq 3.917) = 0.003.$$

Test H_{MT} using
$$q_{(2)} = \max\{0.002, 0.004, 0.003\} = 0.004.$$

(iii) Relevant subsets and their p-values are given by
$$\mathbb{P}(\max\{t_{\mathrm{TV}}, t_{\mathrm{PS}}, t_{\mathrm{MP}}, t_{\mathrm{MS}}\} \geq 3.129) = 0.019 \text{ and}$$
$$\mathbb{P}(\max\{t_{\mathrm{TV}}, t_{\mathrm{PT}}, t_{\mathrm{PV}}, t_{\mathrm{MS}}\} \geq 3.129) = 0.019.$$

Test H_{TV} using
$$q_{(3)} = \max\{0.004, 0.019\} = 0.019.$$

(iv) There is only one relevant subset here, and its p-value is given by
$$\mathbb{P}(\max\{t_{\mathrm{PT}}, t_{\mathrm{SV}}, t_{\mathrm{MV}}, t_{\mathrm{MS}}\} \geq 2.576) = 0.062.$$

Test H_{PT} using
$$q_{(4)} = \max\{0.019, 0.062\} = 0.062.$$

(v) There is only one relevant subset here, and its p-value is given by
$$\mathbb{P}(\max\{t_{\mathrm{PS}}, t_{\mathrm{MP}}, t_{\mathrm{SV}}, t_{\mathrm{MV}}, t_{\mathrm{PV}}, t_{\mathrm{MS}}\} \geq 1.877) = 0.269.$$

Test H_{PS} using
$$q_{(5)} = \max\{0.062, 0.269\} = 0.269.$$

(vi) Relevant subsets and their p-values are given by
$$\mathbb{P}(\max\{t_{MP}, t_{MV}, t_{PV}\} \geq 1.341) = 0.39, \text{ and}$$
$$\mathbb{P}(\max\{t_{MP}, t_{SV}\} \geq 1.341) = 0.347.$$

Test H_{MP} using
$$q_{(6)} = \max\{0.269, 0.39\} = 0.39.$$

(vii) There is only one relevant subset here, and its p-value is given by
$$\mathbb{P}(\max\{t_{SV}, t_{MV}, t_{MS}\} \geq 1.324) = 0.399.$$

Test H_{SV} using
$$q_{(7)} = \max\{0.39, 0.399\} = 0.399.$$

(viii) There is only one relevant subset here, the singleton. Its p-value is given by
$$\mathbb{P}(t_{MV} \geq 0.788) = 0.44,$$
that is, the unadjusted p-value. Test H_{MV} using
$$q_{(8)} = \max\{0.399, 0.44\} = 0.44.$$

(ix) There is only one relevant subset here, and its p-value is given by
$$\mathbb{P}(\max\{t_{PV}, t_{MS}\} \geq 0.553) = 0.826.$$

Test H_{PV} using
$$q_{(9)} = \max\{0.44, 0.826\} = 0.826.$$

(x) There is only one relevant subset here, the singleton. Its p-value is given by
$$\mathbb{P}(t_{MS} \geq 0.536) = 0.598,$$
that is, the unadjusted p-value. Test H_{MS} using
$$q_{(10)} = \max\{0.826, 0.598\} = 0.826.$$

In this example, this is the only case where "truncation" took place, since the adjusted p-value was truncated upward to account for the ordered testing.

Westfall (1997) explained how to automate the process of finding the relevant subsets by using rank conditions involving contrast matrices for the various subsets. In R, truncated closed test procedures are implemented in the **multcomp** package via the `test = adjusted(type = "Westfall")` option. The code below provides exactly the results from the manual calculations above:

```
R> summary(immer.mc, test = adjusted(type = "Westfall"))

        Simultaneous Tests for General Linear Hypotheses

Multiple Comparisons of Means: Tukey Contrasts


Fit: aov(formula = (Y1 + Y2)/2 ~ Var + Loc, data = immer)

Linear Hypotheses:
          Estimate Std. Error t value Pr(>|t|)
P-M == 0      8.15       6.08    1.34   0.3899
S-M == 0     -3.26       6.08   -0.54   0.8257
T-M == 0     23.81       6.08    3.92   0.0045 **
V-M == 0      4.79       6.08    0.79   0.4397
S-P == 0    -11.41       6.08   -1.88   0.2691
T-P == 0     15.66       6.08    2.58   0.0617 .
V-P == 0     -3.36       6.08   -0.55   0.8257
T-S == 0     27.07       6.08    4.45   0.0020 **
V-S == 0      8.05       6.08    1.32   0.3985
V-T == 0    -19.02       6.08   -3.13   0.0192 *
---
Signif. codes:  0 '***' 0.001 '**' 0.01 '*' 0.05 '.' 0.1 ' ' 1
(Adjusted p values reported -- Westfall method)
```

In Table 4.2 we summarize the results from four methods applied to the immer dataset. To be precise, Table 4.2 reports side-by-side the unadjusted p-values p_i from

```
R> summary(immer.mc, test = adjusted(type = "none"))
```

together with the adjusted p-values from the Tukey test, its stepwise extension using truncated closure, and the $S2$ procedure (Shaffer 1986)

```
R> summary(immer.mc, test = adjusted(type = "Shaffer"))
```

The $S2$ procedure differs from type = "Westfall" by using Bonferroni tests instead of the parametric results from Chapter 3. We first conclude that the pairwise comparisons T - M, T - S, and V - T are all significant at level $\alpha = 0.05$, irrespective of which multiple comparison procedure is used. At an unadjusted level, T - P is also significant, although the familywise error rate may not be controlled in this case. Note further, that the truncated closed test procedure from Westfall (1997) – based on max-t tests while exploiting logical constraints and the parametric results from Chapter 3 – leads to uniformly smaller adjusted p-values than both the Tukey test and the Shaffer procedure.

4.3 Dose response analyses

In this section we consider an ANCOVA model for a dose response study with two covariates. In Section 4.3.1 we introduce the example and apply the

Comparison	p_i	Adjusted p-values q_i		
		Tukey	Shaffer	Westfall
P – M	0.195	0.670	0.585	0.390
S – M	0.598	0.982	1.000	0.826
T – M	0.001	0.007	0.005	0.004
V – M	0.440	0.931	0.601	0.440
S – P	0.075	0.361	0.451	0.269
T – P	0.018	0.113	0.072	0.062
V – P	0.587	0.980	1.000	0.826
T – S	0.001	0.002	0.002	0.002
V – S	0.200	0.680	0.601	0.399
V – T	0.005	0.038	0.021	0.019

Table 4.2   Comparison of several multiple comparison procedures for the immer data. Tukey: original Tukey (1953) test (single-step); Shaffer: $S2$ procedure from Shaffer (1986); Westfall: truncated closed test procedure from Westfall (1997).

Dunnett test based on pairwise differences against the control. In Section 4.3.2 we focus on evaluating non-pairwise contrast tests for detecting a dose related trend. In Section 5.3 we extend the disussion and describe related approaches which combine multiple comparison procedures with modeling techniques.

4.3.1 A dose response study on litter weight in mice

Understanding the dose response relationship is a fundamental step in investigating any new compound, whether it is an herbicide or fertilizer, a molecular entity, an environmental toxin, or an industrial chemical (Ruberg 1995a,b; Bretz, Hsu, Pinheiro, and Liu 2008b). For example, determining an adequate dose level for a medicinal drug, and, more broadly, characterizing its dose response relationship with respect to both efficacy and safety, are key objectives of any clinical drug development program. If the dose is set too high, safety and tolerability problems may result, but if the dose is too low it may become difficult to establish adequate efficacy. There is a vast literature on dose finding, especially in the area of pharmaceutical statistics, and we refer the reader to the edited books by Ting (2006); Chevret (2006), and Krishna (2006) for general reading on this topic.

We use a dose response study involving two covariates to illustrate the methods from Chapter 3. Consider the summary statistics in Table 4.3 of a Thalidomide study taken from Westfall and Young (1993) and reanalyzed by Bretz (2006). Four dose levels (0, 5, 50 and 500 units of the study compound) were administered to pregnant mice. Their litters were evaluated for defects and weights. According to Westfall and Young (1993), the primary response variable was the average post-birth weight in the entire litter for the first three weeks of the study. Since the litter weight may depend on gestation time and number of animals in the litter, these two variables were included as covariates in the analysis. We thus consider the ANCOVA model

$$y_{ij} = \beta_0 + \beta_i + \beta_5 z_{1ij} + \beta_6 z_{2ij} + \varepsilon_{ij}, \qquad (4.7)$$

where y_{ij} denotes the weight of the j-th litter at dose level i, z_1 and z_2 the two covariates and $\beta_1, \ldots, \beta_4$ the parameters of interest, namely, the effect of dose level i after adjusting for the effects of the covariates. Finally, the random errors are assumed to be independent, homoscedastic and normally distributed, $\varepsilon_{ij} \sim N(0, \sigma^2)$. Note that model (4.7) is a special case of the general linear model (3.1) and the methods from Section 3.1.1 thus apply to the Thalidomide example. Figure 4.10 displays the covariate-adjusted litter weight data from the Thalidomide study, that is, the least squares means of the four treatment groups together with the associated marginal confidence intervals.

		Dose	0	5	50	500
		Group sample size	20	19	18	17
Weight		Mean	32.31	29.31	29.87	29.65
		Standard deviation	2.70	5.09	3.76	5.40
Gestation time		Mean	22.08	22.21	21.89	22.18
		Standard deviation	0.44	0.45	0.40	0.43
Litter size		Mean	13.40	13.11	14.67	12.53
		Standard deviation	3.02	2.58	1.50	2.58

Table 4.3 Summary data of the Thalidomide dose response example from Westfall and Young (1993).

The experimental question is whether one can claim a statistically significant decrease in average post-birth weight with increasing doses of Thalidomide. A straightforward approach is to perform the pairwise comparisons between the three active dose levels 5, 50, 500 and the zero-dose control, adjusted for covariate effects. In this case the single-step Dunnett test introduced in Section 4.1 is a reasonable approach. To this end, we first fit the ANCOVA model (4.7) to the litter data with the aov function,

```
R> data("litter", package = "multcomp")
R> litter.aov <- aov(weight ~ dose + gesttime + number,
+                    data = litter)
```

and then use the **multcomp** package to perform the Dunnett test,

```
R> litter.mc <- glht(litter.aov, linfct = mcp(dose = "Dunnett"),
+                    alternative = "less")
R> summary(litter.mc, test = adjusted(type = "single-step"))
```

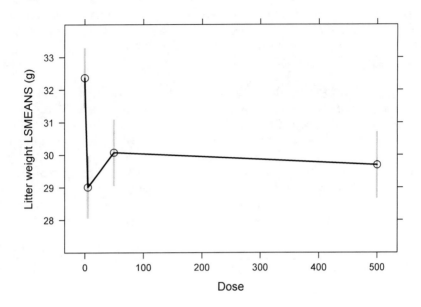

Figure 4.10   Summary plot of the Thalidomide dose response study.

```
      Simultaneous Tests for General Linear Hypotheses

Multiple Comparisons of Means: Dunnett Contrasts


Fit: aov(formula = weight ~ dose + gesttime + number,
  data = litter)

Linear Hypotheses:
             Estimate Std. Error t value Pr(<t)
5 - 0 >= 0     -3.35       1.29    -2.60  0.016 *
50 - 0 >= 0    -2.29       1.34    -1.71  0.112
500 - 0 >= 0   -2.68       1.33    -2.00  0.063 .
---
Signif. codes:  0 '***' 0.001 '**' 0.01 '*' 0.05 '.' 0.1 ' ' 1
(Adjusted p values reported -- single-step method)
```

As seen from the output, the smallest multiplicity adjusted p-value is 0.016. We conclude that there is an overall dose related significant decrease in litter weight. Note that the model fit litter.aov accounts for the two covariates gestation time gesttime and litter size number. The arithmetic means $\bar{y}_i$ and the pooled variance estimate s^2 from the test statistics (4.2) for the Dunnett test in an ANOVA model without covariates have therefore to be replaced by the least squares estimates from the more general expressions (3.3) and (3.4), which also include covariate information. Consequently, the correlations between the test statistics do not follow the simple pattern from Equation (4.3). Using the adjusted(type = "single-step") option in **multcomp** ensures that the stochastic dependencies are all taken into account while performing the closed test procedure, as described in Chapter 3. In addition to the overall significant result, we can assess the adjusted p-values individually. We therefore conclude that the smallest dose level leads to a significant result and the remaining two dose levels lead to only borderline results. We specified alternative = "less" because we are interested in testing for a decreasing trend, that is, whether there was a significant reduction in litter weight.

Note that the more powerful step-down Dunnett test can be applied instead of the single-step Dunnett test by using the adjusted(type = "free") option; see also Section 4.1.2. Using the step-down Dunnett test, the other two dose levels become barely significant: $p = 0.046$ and $p = 0.045$ for the medium and high dose, respectively.

4.3.2 Trend tests

The Dunnett test considered in Section 4.3.1 uses only pairwise comparisons of the individual dose levels with the control. A variety of trend tests have been investigated, which borrow strength from neighboring dose levels when testing for a dose response effect. The approaches proposed by, for example, Bartholomew (1961); Williams (1971), and Marcus (1976) are popular trend tests, which are known to be more powerful than the Dunnett test. However, due to the inclusion of covariates and unequal group sample sizes, these trend tests cannot be applied to the Thalidomide example. In the following we will demonstrate how the framework from Chapter 3 can be applied to the current problem, leading to powerful trend tests for general parametric models.

Consider model (4.7), where the parameter vector $\boldsymbol{\beta}$ consists of $p = 7$ elements β_i. When testing for a dose related trend, one is typically interested in testing the null hypothesis of no treatment effect,

$$H : \beta_1 = \ldots = \beta_4,$$

against the ordered alternative

$$K : \beta_1 \geq \ldots \geq \beta_4 \text{ with } \beta_1 > \beta_4.$$

We conclude in favor of K if the related trend test is significant.

Westfall (1997) proposed the use of three trend contrasts

$$\mathbf{C}_{\text{Westfall}}^{\top} = \begin{pmatrix} 0 & 1.5 & 0.5 & -0.5 & -1.5 & 0 & 0 \\ 0 & 138.75 & 133.75 & 88.75 & -361.25 & 0 & 0 \\ 0 & 0.795 & 0.105 & -0.305 & -0.595 & 0 & 0 \end{pmatrix},$$

to reflect the uncertainty about the underlying dose response shape. The first row of $\mathbf{C}_{\text{Westfall}}^{\top}$ is a simple ordinal trend contrast; the second row is a trend contrast suggested by the arithmetic dose levels; and the third row suggests a log-ordinal dose response relationship. Thus, the use of non-pairwise contrasts allows one to set each of the individual tests into correspondence to some dose response shapes. By using information from all dose levels under investigation, non-pairwise contrast tests tend to be more powerful than the Dunnett test, which is based on pairwise contrasts. Note that in the definition of the matrix $\mathbf{C}_{\text{Westfall}}^{\top}$ the weights for the intercept β_0 and the two covariate parameters β_5 and β_6 are 0, so that the linear function $\mathbf{C}_{\text{Westfall}}^{\top}\boldsymbol{\beta}$ compares only the parameters of interest $\beta_1, \ldots, \beta_4$. In Section 5.3 we will extend these ideas to formally include dose response modeling in a rigid hypotheses testing framework.

The approach from Westfall (1997) sought to let the contrast coefficients mirror potential dose response shapes. Alternatively, the contrast matrix can be specified in a more principled way by reflecting general comparisons among the dose levels, as considered by Williams (1971) and Marcus (1976). Due to the presence of covariates and unequal sample sizes, however, their original approaches cannot be applied to the Thalidomide example. Instead, we follow the proposal of Bretz (2006) and describe the original trend tests of Williams (1971) and Marcus (1976) as contrast tests, so that the results from Chapter 3 are applicable.

We first consider the Williams test extended to the framework of multiple contrast tests. With the sample sizes taken from Table 4.3, the contrast coefficients are given by

$$
\mathbf{C}_{\text{Williams}}^{\top} = \begin{pmatrix} 0 & 1 & 0 & 0 & -1 & 0 & 0 \\ 0 & 1 & 0 & -0.5143 & -0.4857 & 0 & 0 \\ 0 & 1 & -0.3519 & -0.3333 & -0.3148 & 0 & 0 \end{pmatrix}.
$$

Figure 4.11 displays the contrast coefficients for $\beta_1, \ldots, \beta_4$ in the balanced case. Each single contrast test consists of comparisons between the control group and the weighted average over the last ℓ treatment groups, $\ell = 1, \ldots, 3$, respectively. To illustrate this, consider the second row of $\mathbf{C}_{\text{Williams}}^{\top}$. The control group is compared with the weighted average of the two highest dose levels. The weight for the control group is 1. The weights for the highest and second highest dose levels are $-17/(17+18) = -0.4857$ and $-18/(17+18) = -0.5143$, respectively; here, 17 and 18 are the respective group sample sizes taken from Table 4.3. The lowest dose level is not included in this comparison and is therefore assigned the weight 0. Note that the weights for the intercept β_0 and the two covariate parameters β_5 and β_6 are set to 0, so that $\mathbf{C}_{\text{Williams}}^{\top}\boldsymbol{\beta}$ involves only the comparison of the parameters of interest. As shown by Bretz (2006), using the matrix $\mathbf{C}_{\text{Williams}}^{\top}$ ensures that the same type of comparison is performed as with the original test of Williams (1971) while taking into account the information of the covariates through the computation of the least squares estimates $\hat{\boldsymbol{\beta}}$ and $\hat{\sigma}$.

We can compute the contrast matrix $\mathbf{C}_{\text{Williams}}^{\top}$ with the contrMat function from the **multcomp** package. This function computes the contrast matrices

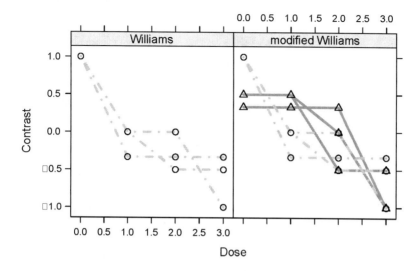

Figure 4.11   Plot of contrast coefficients for the Williams test (left, dot dashed
lines with circles) and the modified Williams test (right, solid lines
with triangles and dot dashed lines with circles), in the balanced
case.

for several multiple comparison procedures, including, among others, the tests
of Dunnett and Tukey, as well as the trend tests of Williams and Marcus
(contrast version). Its syntax is straightforward and we obtain the contrast
matrix $\mathbf{C}^{\top}_{\text{Williams}}$ with the statements

```
R> n <- c(20, 19, 18, 17)
R> -contrMat(n, type = "Williams")
```

    Multiple Comparisons of Means: Williams Contrasts

```
      1      2        3       4
C 1  1   0.000   0.000  -1.000
C 2  1   0.000  -0.514  -0.486
C 3  1  -0.352  -0.333  -0.315
```

Note that `contrMat` computes the contrast coefficients under the assumption
of an increasing trend. In the Thalidomide example we are interested in detecting a reduction in litter weight and therefore the resulting coefficients from
`contrMat` need to be multiplied by -1.

  The modified Williams test (Williams 1971; Marcus 1976) can be extended similarly and the corresponding contrast coefficients are given by

$$
\mathbf{C}_{\text{mod Williams}}^{\top} = \begin{pmatrix}
0 & 1 & 0 & 0 & -1 & 0 & 0 \\
0 & 1 & 0 & -0.5143 & -0.4857 & 0 & 0 \\
0 & 1 & -0.3519 & -0.3333 & -0.3148 & 0 & 0 \\
0 & 0.5128 & 0.4872 & -0.5143 & -0.4857 & 0 & 0 \\
0 & 0.5128 & 0.4872 & 0 & -1 & 0 & 0 \\
0 & 0.3509 & 0.3333 & 0.3158 & -1 & 0 & 0
\end{pmatrix}.
$$

Figure 4.11 also plots the coefficients for the contrast version of the modified Williams test. Note that $\mathbf{C}_{\text{Williams}}^{\top}$ is a subset of $\mathbf{C}_{\text{mod Williams}}^{\top}$ in the sense that the weights for the former test are all contained in the contrast matrix of the latter test (the first three rows). These weights are particularly suitable for testing concave dose response shapes, as the higher dose groups are pooled and compared with the zero dose group. The rows five and six of $\mathbf{C}_{\text{mod Williams}}^{\top}$ are appropriate for detecting convex shapes, as they average the lower treatments. The fourth row is particularly powerful for linear or approximately linear relationships. To illustrate the computation of the coefficients for the fourth contrast, we note that the weighted average of the two higher dose levels is compared with the weighted average of the remaining treatments. With the group sample sizes taken from Table 4.3, we therefore obtain $20/(20 + 19) = 0.5128, 19/(20 + 19) = 0.4872, 18/(18 + 17) = 0.5143$, and $17/(18 + 17) = 0.4857$. We refer to Bretz (2006) for the analytical expressions of the contrast coefficients in general linear models. Using the contrMat function, we can compute $\mathbf{C}_{\text{mod Williams}}^{\top}$ with the call

```
R> -contrMat(n, type = "Marcus")
```

```
     Multiple Comparisons of Means: Marcus Contrasts


          1       2       3       4
C 1   1.000  -0.352  -0.333  -0.315
C 2   1.000   0.000  -0.514  -0.486
C 3   0.513   0.487  -0.514  -0.486
C 4   1.000   0.000   0.000  -1.000
C 5   0.513   0.487   0.000  -1.000
C 6   0.351   0.333   0.316  -1.000
```

We now illustrate, how the **multcomp** package can be used to analyze the Thalidomide example with the contrast versions of the trend tests from Williams (1971) and Marcus (1976). Similar to what was done in Section 4.3.1, we can apply the glht function to the fitted aov object. In order to perform the Williams contrast test we pass the mcp(dose = "Williams") option to the linfct argument,

```
R> litter.mc2 <- glht(litter.aov, alternative = "less",
+                     linfct = mcp(dose = "Williams"))
R> summary(litter.mc2)
```

```
     Simultaneous Tests for General Linear Hypotheses
```

Multiple Comparisons of Means: Williams Contrasts


```
Fit: aov(formula = weight ~ dose + gesttime + number,
   data = litter)
```

```
Linear Hypotheses:
           Estimate Std. Error t value Pr(<t)
C 1 >= 0    -2.68       1.33     -2.00  0.0436 *
C 2 >= 0    -2.48       1.12     -2.21  0.0285 *
C 3 >= 0    -2.79       1.05     -2.66  0.0097 **
---
```

Signif. codes: 0 '***' 0.001 '**' 0.01 '*' 0.05 '.' 0.1 ' ' 1
(Adjusted p values reported -- single-step method)

The adjusted p-value for the Williams contrast test is the minimum of the set of three p-values listed in the last column. In our example, the adjusted p-value is 0.01 and we conclude for a significant dose response signal at the 5% significance level. Note that this p-value is smaller than the adjusted p-value 0.016 for the Dunnett test from Section 4.3.1. This indicates that trend tests indeed tend to be more powerful than the pairwise comparisons from Dunnett. In analogy to the previous glht call, we can also apply the modified Williams test by calling

```
R> glht(litter.aov, linfct = mcp(dose = "Marcus"),
+       alternative = "less")
```

We can improve the Williams test by applying the closure principle from Section 2.2.3. Technically, the $m = 3$ elementary one-sided hypotheses are given by $H_j : \mathbf{c}_j^\top \boldsymbol{\beta} \leq 0$, where $\boldsymbol{\beta}$ denotes the 7×1 parameter vector introduced in Section 4.3.1 and $\mathbf{c}_j^\top$ is the j-th row of $\mathbf{C}_{\text{Williams}}^\top$, $j = 1, 2, 3$. Note that the contrast coefficients have been scaled such that large values of $\mathbf{c}_j^\top \boldsymbol{\beta}$ indicate a dose related weight loss. With the closure principle, we consider in addition all pairwise intersection hypotheses $H_i \cap H_j$, $1 = i < j = 3$, and the global intersection null hypothesis $H_1 \cap H_2 \cap H_3$. The Williams contrasts satisfy the free combination property (Section 2.1.2), because there is one additional free parameter in each successive contrast. We can thus apply the mcp(dose = "free") option discussed in Section 4.1.2,

```
R> summary(litter.mc2, test = adjusted(type = "free"))
```

Simultaneous Tests for General Linear Hypotheses

Multiple Comparisons of Means: Williams Contrasts


```
Fit: aov(formula = weight ~ dose + gesttime + number,
   data = litter)
```

```
Linear Hypotheses:
          Estimate Std. Error t value Pr(<t)
C 1 >= 0     -2.68      1.33   -2.00 0.0245 *
C 2 >= 0     -2.48      1.12   -2.21 0.0237 *
C 3 >= 0     -2.79      1.05   -2.66 0.0091 **
---
Signif. codes:  0 '***' 0.001 '**' 0.01 '*' 0.05 '.' 0.1 ' ' 1
(Adjusted p values reported -- free method)
```

As seen from the output, the application of the closure principle leads to a reduction of the adjusted p-values.

4.4 Variable selection in regression models

Garcia, Wagner, Hothorn, Koebnick, Zunft, and Trippo (2005) applied predictive regression equations to body fat content with nine common anthropometric measurements, which were obtained from 71 healthy German women. In addition, the body composition was measured by Dual Energy X-Ray Absorptiometry (DXA). This reference method is very accurate in measuring body fat but has limited practical application because of its high costs and challenging methodology. Therefore, a simple regression equation for predicting DXA body fat measurements is of special interest for the practitioner. Backward-elimination was applied to select important variables from the available anthropometrical measurements. Garcia et al. (2005) reported a final linear model utilizing hip circumference, knee breadth and a compound covariate defined as the sum of the logarithmized chin, triceps and subscapular skinfolds.

Here, we fit the saturated model to the data and use adjusted p-values to select important variables, where the multiplicity adjustment accounts for the correlation between the test statistics; see Chapter 3. We use the lm function such that the linear model including all covariates with the unadjusted p-values is given by

```
R> data("bodyfat", package = "mboost")
R> bodyfat.lm <- lm(DEXfat ~ ., data = bodyfat)
R> summary(bodyfat.lm)
```

```
Call:
lm(formula = DEXfat ~ ., data = bodyfat)

Residuals:
   Min     1Q Median     3Q    Max
-6.954 -1.949 -0.219  1.169 10.812

Coefficients:
            Estimate Std. Error t value Pr(>|t|)
(Intercept) -69.0283     7.5169   -9.18 4.2e-13 ***
age           0.0200     0.0322    0.62  0.5378
waistcirc     0.2105     0.0671    3.13  0.0026 **
```

```
hipcirc            0.3435      0.0804     4.27   6.9e-05 ***
elbowbreadth      -0.4124      1.0229    -0.40   0.6883
kneebreadth        1.7580      0.7250     2.42   0.0183 *
anthro3a           5.7423      5.2075     1.10   0.2745
anthro3b           9.8664      5.6579     1.74   0.0862 .
anthro3c           0.3874      2.0875     0.19   0.8534
anthro4           -6.5744      6.4892    -1.01   0.3150
---
Signif. codes:  0 '***' 0.001 '**' 0.01 '*' 0.05 '.' 0.1 ' ' 1

Residual standard error: 3.28 on 61 degrees of freedom
Multiple R-squared: 0.923,        Adjusted R-squared: 0.912
F-statistic: 81.3 on 9 and 61 DF,  p-value: <2e-16
```

The matrix **C**, which defines the experimental questions of interest, is essentially the identity matrix, except for the intercept, which is omitted. This reflects our interest in assessing each individual variable:

```
R> K <- cbind(0, diag(length(coef(bodyfat.lm)) - 1))
R> rownames(K) <- names(coef(bodyfat.lm))[-1]
R> K
```

```
             [,1] [,2] [,3] [,4] [,5] [,6] [,7] [,8] [,9] [,10]
age             0    1    0    0    0    0    0    0    0     0
waistcirc       0    0    1    0    0    0    0    0    0     0
hipcirc         0    0    0    1    0    0    0    0    0     0
elbowbreadth    0    0    0    0    1    0    0    0    0     0
kneebreadth     0    0    0    0    0    1    0    0    0     0
anthro3a        0    0    0    0    0    0    1    0    0     0
anthro3b        0    0    0    0    0    0    0    1    0     0
anthro3c        0    0    0    0    0    0    0    0    1     0
anthro4         0    0    0    0    0    0    0    0    0     1
```

Once the matrix **C** is defined, it can be used to set up the multiple comparison problem using the `glht` function in **multcomp**

```
R> bodyfat.mc <- glht(bodyfat.lm, linfct = K)
```

Traditionally, one would perform an F test to check if any of the regression coefficients is significant,

```
R> summary(bodyfat.mc, test = Ftest())
```

```
            General Linear Hypotheses

Linear Hypotheses:
                        Estimate
age == 0                  0.0200
waistcirc == 0            0.2105
hipcirc == 0              0.3435
elbowbreadth == 0        -0.4124
kneebreadth == 0          1.7580
anthro3a == 0             5.7423
```

```
anthro3b == 0          9.8664
anthro3c == 0          0.3874
anthro4 == 0          -6.5744


Global Test:
     F DF1 DF2    Pr(>F)
1 81.3    9   61 1.39e-30
```

As seen from the output, the F test is highly significant. However, because the F test is an omnibus test, we cannot assess which covariates significantly deviate from 0 while controlling the familywise error rate. Calculating the individual adjusted p-values provides the necessary information,

```
R> summary(bodyfat.mc)
```

```
       Simultaneous Tests for General Linear Hypotheses

Fit: lm(formula = DEXfat ~ ., data = bodyfat)

Linear Hypotheses:
                   Estimate Std. Error t value Pr(>|t|)
age == 0             0.0200     0.0322    0.62    0.996
waistcirc == 0       0.2105     0.0671    3.13    0.022 *
hipcirc == 0         0.3435     0.0804    4.27   <0.001 ***
elbowbreadth == 0   -0.4124     1.0229   -0.40    1.000
kneebreadth == 0     1.7580     0.7250    2.42    0.132
anthro3a == 0        5.7423     5.2075    1.10    0.895
anthro3b == 0        9.8664     5.6579    1.74    0.478
anthro3c == 0        0.3874     2.0875    0.19    1.000
anthro4 == 0        -6.5744     6.4892   -1.01    0.930
---
Signif. codes:  0 '***' 0.001 '**' 0.01 '*' 0.05 '.' 0.1 ' ' 1
(Adjusted p values reported -- single-step method)
```

We conclude that only two covariates, `waist` and `hip` circumference, seem to be relevant and contribute to the significant F test. Note that this conclusion is drawn while controlling the familywise error rate in the strong sense; see Section 2.1.1 for a description of suitable error rates in multiple hypotheses testing.

Alternatively, MM-estimates (Yohai 1987) can be applied and we can use the results from Section 3.2 to perform suitable multiple comparisons for the robustified linear model. We use the `lmrob` function from the **robustbase** package (Rousseeuw, Croux, Todorov, Ruckstuhl, Salibian-Barrera, Verbeke, and Maechler 2009) to fit a robust version of the previous linear model. Interestingly enough, the results coincide rather nicely,

```
R> vcov.lmrob <-function(object) object$cov
R> summary(glht(lmrob(DEXfat ~ ., data = bodyfat),
+                linfct = K))
```

```
       Simultaneous Tests for General Linear Hypotheses
```

```
Fit: lmrob(formula = DEXfat ~ ., data = bodyfat)
```

```
Linear Hypotheses:
                   Estimate Std. Error z value Pr(>|z|)
age == 0             0.0264     0.0193    1.37   0.7242
waistcirc == 0       0.2318     0.0665    3.49   0.0041 **
hipcirc == 0         0.3293     0.0755    4.36   <0.001 ***
elbowbreadth == 0   -0.2549     0.9245   -0.28   1.0000
kneebreadth == 0     0.7738     0.5280    1.47   0.6523
anthro3a == 0        2.0706     3.6597    0.57   0.9974
anthro3b == 0       10.1589     4.7770    2.13   0.2190
anthro3c == 0        1.9133     1.4040    1.36   0.7262
anthro4 == 0        -5.6737     5.5795   -1.02   0.9194
---
Signif. codes:  0 '***' 0.001 '**' 0.01 '*' 0.05 '.' 0.1 ' ' 1
(Adjusted p values reported -- single-step method)
```

4.5 Simultaneous confidence bands for the comparison of two linear regression models

Kleinbaum, Kupper, Muller, and Nizam (1998) considered how systolic blood pressure changes with age for both females and males. From the data they have collected it is clear that the relationship between systolic blood pressure y and age x can be reasonably described by a linear regression model of y on x for both gender groups. A natural question is whether the two linear regression models for female and male are the same. That is, we want to compare the two linear regression models for a continuous range of a covariate x (that is, age in our example).

Let

$$y_{ij} = \beta_{0i} + \beta_{1i}x_{ij} + \varepsilon_{ij} \qquad (4.8)$$

denote two simple linear regression models, one for females $(i = F)$ and one for males $(i = M)$. Each gender has its own regression parameters, the intercept β_{0i} and the slope β_{1i}. In Equation (4.8), the index j denotes the j-th observation (within gender $i = F, M$). Finally, we assume independent and normally distributed residuals $\varepsilon_{ij} \sim N(0, \sigma^2)$. In the matrix notation from Section 3.1, model (4.8) can be written as $\mathbf{y}_i = \mathbf{X}_i\boldsymbol{\beta}_i + \boldsymbol{\varepsilon}_i, i = F, M$.

The frequently used approach to the problem of comparing two linear regression models is to use an F test for the null hypothesis $H: \boldsymbol{\beta}_1 = \boldsymbol{\beta}_2$. If H is rejected then the two regression models are deemed different. Otherwise, if H is not rejected, then there is insufficient statistical evidence to conclude the two regression models are different. But no tangible information on the magnitude of the difference between the two models is provided by this hypotheses testing approach, whether H is rejected or not. For instance, in the example from Kleinbaum et al. (1998) the p-value for the F test is less than 0.0001 and so there is a strong statistical indication that the two regression models are different. But no measurement is provided for the degree of difference between these two regression models.

Following Liu, Jamshidian, Zhang, Bretz, and Han (2007a), we now discuss the construction of a two-sided *simultaneous confidence band* as a more intuitive alternative to the F test. The null hypothesis H is rejected if the $y = 0$ line does not lie completely inside the confidence band. The advantage of this confidence band approach over the F test is that it provides information on the magnitude of the difference between the two regression models, whether or not H is rejected.

Note that in practice we often have linear regression models that are of interest only over a restricted region of the covariates. In the systolic blood pressure example above, it is natural to exclude negative x ($=$ age) values and perhaps restrict the range for x even further. The part of the confidence band outside this restricted region is useless for inference. It is therefore unnecessary to guarantee the $1 - \alpha$ simultaneous coverage probability over the entire range of the covariate. Furthermore, inferences deduced from the confidence band outside the restricted region, such as the rejection of H, may not be valid since the assumed model may be wrong outside the restricted region. This calls for the construction of a $1 - \alpha$ simultaneous confidence band over a restricted region of the covariate. Note that unlike other applications covered in this book, this is an example of inferences for infinite sets of linear functions. Because we test for each single $x \in [a, b]$, say, whether the two regression models are the same, we have an infinite number of hypotheses.

The simultaneous confidence band to be constructed is of the form

$$\mathbf{x}^\top \boldsymbol{\beta}_1 - \mathbf{x}^\top \boldsymbol{\beta}_2 \in \left[\mathbf{x}^\top \hat{\boldsymbol{\beta}}_1 - \mathbf{x}^\top \hat{\boldsymbol{\beta}}_2 \pm u_{1-\alpha} s \sqrt{\mathbf{x}^\top \boldsymbol{\Delta} \mathbf{x}} \right],$$

where $\mathbf{x} = (1, x)^\top$, $x \in [a, b]$, $\boldsymbol{\Delta} = (\mathbf{X}_1^\top \mathbf{X}_1)^{-1} + (\mathbf{X}_2^\top \mathbf{X}_2)^{-1}$, and s^2 denotes the pooled variance estimate. The construction of the simultaneous confidence bands depends on the critical value $u_{1-\alpha}$. In order to ensure a simultaneous coverage probability of at least $1 - \alpha$, the critical value $u_{1-\alpha}$ is chosen such that $\mathbb{P}(t_{\max} \leq u_{1-\alpha}) = 1 - \alpha$, where

$$t_{\max} = \sup_{x \in [a,b]} \frac{|\mathbf{x}^\top [(\hat{\boldsymbol{\beta}}_1 - \boldsymbol{\beta}_1) - (\hat{\boldsymbol{\beta}}_2 - \boldsymbol{\beta}_2)]|}{s \sqrt{\mathbf{x}^\top \boldsymbol{\Delta} \mathbf{x}}}. \tag{4.9}$$

Because in the present case the distribution of $t_{\max}$ is not available in closed form, efficient simulations methods have to be used to calculate the critical value $u_{1-\alpha}$. Liu et al. (2007a), extending earlier methods from Liu, Jamshidian, and Zhang (2004), suggested simulating a large number of times, R say, replicates of the random variable $t_{\max}$ from (4.9) and take the $(1 - \alpha)R$-th largest simulated value as the critical values $u_{1-\alpha}$.

The method of Liu et al. (2007a) is rather complex and requires special software implementations. Here, we approximate the critical value $u_{1-\alpha}$ by discretizing the covariate region $[a, b]$. That is, instead of considering the supremum over the continuous interval $[a, b]$ in (4.9), we suggest considering the maximum over the equally spaced values $a = x_1 < x_2 < \ldots < x_k = b$; see also Westfall et al. (1999) for a related approach to construct simultaneous confidence bands for a single linear regression model. The resulting critical value should be very close to the correct one when k is large.

The advantage of this approach is that one can use the **multcomp** package for the necessary calculations. Suppose we fit linear regression models for both gender with the lm function to the sbp data from Kleinbaum et al. (1998)

```
R> data("sbp", package = "multcomp")
R> sbp.lm <- lm(sbp ~ gender * age, data = sbp)
R> coef(sbp.lm)
```

```
    (Intercept)        genderfemale                    age
       110.0385            -12.9614                 0.9614
genderfemale:age
        -0.0120
```

We then define a grid for the covariate region, thereby defining the linear functions, by calling

```
R> age <- seq(from = 17, to = 47, by = 1)
R> K <- cbind(0, 1, 0, age)
R> rownames(K) <- paste("age", age, sep = "")
```

Finally, we call the glht function and obtain an approximate 99% simultaneous confidence band with

```
R> sbp.mc <- glht(sbp.lm, linfct = K)
R> sbp.ci <- confint(sbp.mc, level = 0.99)
```

Note that the resulting critical value is

```
R> attr(sbp.ci$confint, "calpha")
```

```
[1] 2.97
```

which is very close to the value $u_{1-\alpha} = 2.969$ obtained by Liu et al. (2007a) based on $R = 1,000,000$ simulations using their sophisticated method. The resulting confidence band can be plotted using

```
R> plot(age, coef(sbp.mc), type = "l", ylim = c(-30, 2))
R> lines(age, sbp.ci$confint[,"upr"])
R> lines(age, sbp.ci$confint[,"lwr"])
R> abline(h = 0, lty = 2)
```

It follows from Figure 4.12 that H is rejected (at $\alpha = 0.01$) because the $y = 0$ line is not included in the band for any $20 \le x \le 47$. Furthermore, one can infer from the band that females tend to have significantly lower blood pressure than males between the ages of 20 and 47, because the upper curve of the band lies below the zero line for $20 \le x \le 47$. This inference cannot be made from the F test, because it does not provide information beyond whether or not two regression models are the same. This illustrates the advantage of using a simultaneous confidence band instead of the F test.

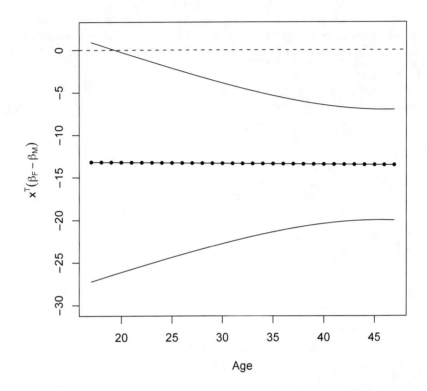

Figure 4.12   Simultaneous confidence band for the difference of two linear regression models over the observed range $17 \leq$ age ≤ 47 for the sbp data
($\alpha = 0.01$).

We conclude this example by noting that the approximation methods presented here can be extended easily using **multcomp** to accommodate more
than one covariate, construct one-sided simultaneous confidence bands, and
derive simultaneous confidence bands for other types of applications, such as
a single linear regression model. We refer to Liu (2010) for details on exact
simultaneous inference in regression models.

4.6 Multiple comparisons under heteroscedasticity

Various studies have linked alcohol dependence phenotypes to chromosome
4. One candidate gene is *NACP* (non-amyloid component of plaques), cod-
ing for alpha synuclein. Bönsch, Lederer, Reulbach, Hothorn, Kornhuber, and
Bleich (2005) found longer alleles of *NACP*-REP1 in alcohol-dependent pa-

tients compared with healthy volunteers. They reported that allele lengths show some association with the expression level alpha synuclein mRNA in alcohol-dependent subjects (see Figure 4.13). Allele length is measured as a summary score from additive dinucleotide repeat length and categorized into three groups: short $(0 - 4, n = 24$ subjects), medium $(5 - 9, n = 58)$, and long $(10 - 12, n = 15)$. Here, we are interested in comparing the mean expression level of alpha synuclein mRNA in the three groups of subjects defined by allele length.

To start with, we load the dataset,

```
R> data("alpha", package = "coin")
```

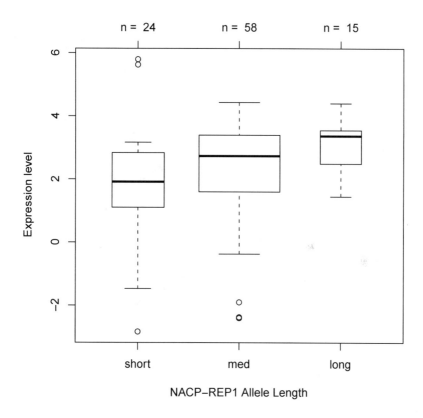

Figure 4.13   Distribution of expression levels for alpha synuclein mRNA in three groups defined by the *NACP*-REP1 allele lengths.

fit a simple one-way ANOVA model to the data with the **aov** function

```
R> alpha.aov <- aov(elevel ~ alength, data = alpha)
```

and apply the (single-step) Tukey test using the `glht` function in **multcomp**

```
R> alpha.mc <- glht(alpha.aov, linfct = mcp(alength = "Tukey"))
```

We therefore let the contrast matrix, which defines the experimental questions of interest, contain all pairwise differences between the three groups and use the `mcp(alength = "Tukey")` option for the `linfct` argument; see Section 4.2 for a detailed description of the Tukey test.

As explained in Section 3.3.1, the default in R to fit ANOVA and regression models is using a suitable reparametrization of the parameter vector based on the so-called treatment contrasts. The first group is treated as a control group, with which the other groups are compared. Accordingly, the contrast matrix accounting for the reparametrization is given by

```
R> alpha.mc$linfct
```

```
              (Intercept) alengthmed alengthlong
med - short         0          1           0
long - short        0          0           1
long - med          0         -1           1
attr(,"type")
[1] "Tukey"
```

With the framework of model (3.1) we obtain all pairwise comparisons of the mean expression levels through

$$
\begin{pmatrix} 0 & 1 & 0 \\ 0 & 0 & 1 \\ 0 & -1 & 1 \end{pmatrix} \begin{pmatrix} \beta_0 \\ \beta_2 - \beta_1 \\ \beta_3 - \beta_1 \end{pmatrix} = \begin{pmatrix} \beta_2 - \beta_1 \\ \beta_3 - \beta_1 \\ \beta_3 - \beta_2 \end{pmatrix},
$$

where β_0 denotes the intercept and β_i denotes the mean effect of group $i = 1, 2, 3$.

The `alpha.mc` object also contains information about the estimated linear functions of interest and the associated covariance matrix. These quantities can be retrieved with the `coef` and `vcov` methods:

```
R> coef(alpha.mc)
```

```
 med - short long - short   long - med
       0.434        1.189        0.755
```

```
R> vcov(alpha.mc)
```

```
              med - short long - short long - med
med - short        0.1472       0.104     -0.0431
long - short       0.1041       0.271      0.1666
long - med        -0.0431       0.167      0.2096
```

The `summary` and `confint` methods can be used to compute the summary statistics, including adjusted p-values and simultaneous confidence intervals,

```
R> confint(alpha.mc)
```

Simultaneous Confidence Intervals

Multiple Comparisons of Means: Tukey Contrasts

Fit: aov(formula = elevel ~ alength, data = alpha)

Quantile = 2.37
95% family-wise confidence level

Linear Hypotheses:
```
                 Estimate  lwr      upr
med  - short == 0  0.4342  -0.4758  1.3441
long - short == 0  1.1888  -0.0452  2.4227
long - med   == 0  0.7546  -0.3314  1.8406
```

R> summary(alpha.mc)

Simultaneous Tests for General Linear Hypotheses

Multiple Comparisons of Means: Tukey Contrasts

Fit: aov(formula = elevel ~ alength, data = alpha)

Linear Hypotheses:
```
                 Estimate  Std. Error  t value  Pr(>|t|)
med  - short == 0   0.434     0.384      1.13    0.492
long - short == 0   1.189     0.520      2.28    0.061 .
long - med   == 0   0.755     0.458      1.65    0.227
---
```
Signif. codes: 0 '***' 0.001 '**' 0.01 '*' 0.05 '.' 0.1 ' ' 1
(Adjusted p values reported -- single-step method)

From this output we conclude that there is no significant difference between any combination of the three allele lengths.

Looking at Figure 4.13, however, the variance homogeneity assumption is questionable and one might challenge the validity of these results. One may argue that a sandwich estimate is more appropriate in this situation. Based on the results from Section 3.2, we use the **sandwich** function from the **sandwich** package (Zeileis 2006), which provides a heteroscedasticity-consistent estimate of the covariance matrix. The **vcov** argument of **glht** can be used to specify the alternative estimate,

```
R> alpha.mc2 <- glht(alpha.aov, linfct = mcp(alength = "Tukey"),
+                      vcov = sandwich)
R> summary(alpha.mc2)
```

Simultaneous Tests for General Linear Hypotheses

Multiple Comparisons of Means: Tukey Contrasts

Fit: aov(formula = elevel ~ alength, data = alpha)

Linear Hypotheses:

	Estimate	Std. Error	t value	Pr(>|t|)
med - short == 0	0.434	0.424	1.02	0.559
long - short == 0	1.189	0.443	2.68	0.023 *
long - med == 0	0.755	0.318	2.37	0.050 .

---
*Signif. codes: 0 '***' 0.001 '**' 0.01 '*' 0.05 '.' 0.1 ' ' 1*
(Adjusted p values reported -- single-step method)

Now, having applied the sandwich estimate, the group with long allele lengths is significantly different from the other two groups at the 5% significance level. This result matches previously published study results based on non-parametric analyses. A comparison of the simultaneous confidence intervals based on the ordinary estimate of the covariance matrix and the sandwich estimate is given in Figure 4.14.

4.7 Multiple comparisons in logistic regression models

Salib and Hillier (1997) reported the results of a case-control study to investigate Alzheimer's disease and smoking behavior of 198 female and male Alzheimer patients and 164 controls. The Alzheimer data shown in Table 4.4 have been reconstructed from Table 4 in Salib and Hillier (1997) and are depicted in Figure 4.15; see also Hothorn, Hornik, van de Wiel, and Zeileis (2006). Originally, the authors were interested in assessing whether there is any association between smoking and Alzheimer's diseases (or other types of dementia). After analyzing the study data, they concluded that cigarette smoking is less frequent in men with Alzheimer's disease. In this section we describe how a potential association can be investigated in subgroup analyses using suitable multiple comparison procedures.

In what follows below we consider a logistic regression model with the two factors **gender** (male and female) and **smoking**. Smoking habit was classified into four levels, depending on daily cigarette consumption: no smoking, less than 10, between 10 and 20, and more than 20 cigarettes per day. The response is a binary variable describing the diagnosis of the patient (either suffering or not from Alzheimer's disease). Using the **glm** function, we fit a logistic regression model that includes both main effects and an interaction effect of **smoking** and **gender**,

Ordinary covariance matrix estimate

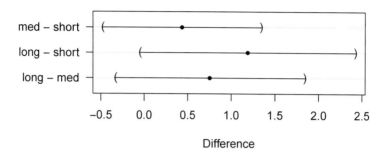

Sandwich estimate

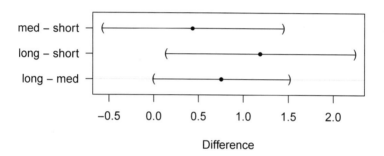

Figure 4.14 Simultaneous confidence intervals based on the ordinary estimate of the covariance matrix (top) and a sandwich estimate (bottom).

```
R> data("alzheimer", package = "coin")
R> y <- factor(alzheimer$disease == "Alzheimer",
+              labels = c("other", "Alzheimer"))
R> alzheimer.glm <- glm(y ~ smoking * gender,
+       data = alzheimer, family = binomial())
```

and use the summary method associated with the glht function to get a detailed output:

```
R> summary(alzheimer.glm)
```

```
Call:
glm(formula = y ~ smoking * gender, family = binomial(),
    data = alzheimer)

Deviance Residuals:
```

	No. of cigarettes daily			
	None	<10	10–20	>20
Female				
Alzheimer	91	7	15	21
Other dementias	55	7	16	9
Other diagnoses	80	3	25	9
Male				
Alzheimer	35	8	15	6
Other dementias	24	1	17	35
Other diagnoses	24	2	22	11

Table 4.4   Summary of the `alzheimer` data.

```
    Min      1Q   Median      3Q     Max
  -1.61   -1.02    -0.79    1.31    2.08

Coefficients:
                        Estimate Std. Error z value Pr(>|z|)
(Intercept)              -0.3944     0.1356   -2.91  0.00364
smoking<10                0.0377     0.5111    0.07  0.94114
smoking10-20             -0.6111     0.3308   -1.85  0.06473
smoking>20                0.5486     0.3487    1.57  0.11565
genderMale                0.0786     0.2604    0.30  0.76287
smoking<10:genderMale     1.2589     0.8769    1.44  0.15111
smoking10-20:genderMale  -0.0286     0.5012   -0.06  0.95457
smoking>20:genderMale    -2.2696     0.5995   -3.79  0.00015

(Dispersion parameter for binomial family taken to be 1)

    Null deviance: 707.90  on 537  degrees of freedom
Residual deviance: 673.55  on 530  degrees of freedom
AIC: 689.5

Number of Fisher Scoring iterations: 4
```

The negative regression coefficient for males who are heavy smokers indicates that Alzheimer's disease might be less frequent in this group. But the model remains difficult to interpret based on the coefficients and corresponding p-values only. Therefore, we compute simultaneous confidence intervals on the probability scale for the different risk groups. For each factor combination of gender and smoking, the probability of suffering from Alzheimer's disease can be estimated by computing the logit function of the linear predictor from the `alzheimer.glm` model fit. Using the `predict` method for generalized linear models is a convenient way to compute these probability estimates. Alterna-

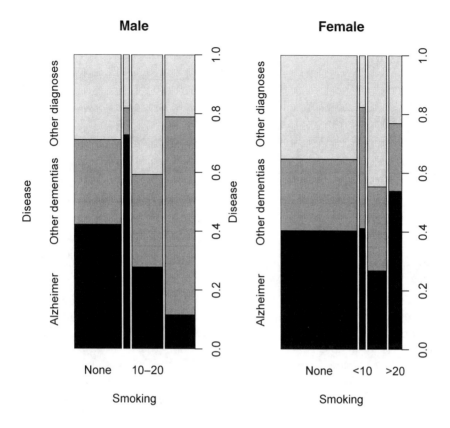

Figure 4.15 Association between smoking behavior and disease status stratified by gender.

tively, we can set up a matrix $\mathbf{C}$ such that, in the notation from Section 3.2,

$$\frac{1}{1 + \exp(-\hat{\boldsymbol{\vartheta}}_n)}$$

is the vector of estimated probabilities with simultaneous confidence intervals

$$\left[\frac{1}{1 + \exp\left(-\left(\hat{\boldsymbol{\vartheta}}_n - u_{1-\alpha} \mathrm{diag}(\mathbf{D})_n^{1/2} \right) \right)}; \right. \tag{4.10}$$

$$\left. \frac{1}{1 + \exp\left(-\left(\hat{\boldsymbol{\vartheta}}_n + u_{1-\alpha} \mathrm{diag}(\mathbf{D})_n^{1/2} \right) \right)} \right].$$

In our model, $\mathbf{C}$ is given by

```
R> K
```

	(Icpt)	s<10	s10-20	s>20	gMale	s<10:gMale
None:Female	1	0	0	0	0	0
<10:Female	1	1	0	0	0	0
10-20:Female	1	0	1	0	0	0
>20:Female	1	0	0	1	0	0
None:Male	1	0	0	0	1	0
<10:Male	1	1	0	0	1	1
10-20:Male	1	0	1	0	1	0
>20:Male	1	0	0	1	1	0

	s10-20:gMale	s>20:gMale
None:Female	0	0
<10:Female	0	0
10-20:Female	0	0
>20:Female	0	0
None:Male	0	0
<10:Male	0	0
10-20:Male	1	0
>20:Male	0	1

where the rows represent the eight factor combinations of **gender** and **smoking** and the columns match the parameter vector. Recall from Section 3.3.1 that the default in R to fit ANOVA and regression models is using a suitable re-parametrization of the parameter vector based on the so-called treatment contrasts. In the **alzheimer** example, the non-smoking female group **None:Female** is treated as a common reference group, to which the other groups are compared. For example, to obtain the effect **<10:Male** of males smoking less than 10 cigarettes, we need to add the female effect **s<10** of smoking less than 10 cigarettes, the male gender effect **gMale** and their interaction effect **s<10:gMale**. Thus, row 6 in the matrix above has the entries 1 in the associated columns and 0 otherwise. The other seven rows are interpreted similarly.

Having set up the matrix **C** this way, we can call

```
R> alzheimer.ci <- confint(glht(alzheimer.glm, linfct = K))
```

where

```
R> attr(alzheimer.ci$confint, "calpha")
```

[1] 2.73

gives the critical value from the joint asymptotic multivariate normal distribution. Note, however, that we have eight factor combinations with independent patients. The test statistics are therefore uncorrelated as long as no covariates are included in the analysis. The Šidák approach described in Section 2.3.3 is exact in this situation and the critical value above can also be obtained by calling

```
R> qnorm((1-(1-0.05)^(1/8))/2, lower.tail = FALSE)
```

[1] 2.73

This example shows that although **multcomp** always gives correct results, it can be replaced by more efficient direct approaches in special situations.

Finally, we can compute the simultaneous confidence intervals (4.10) and plot them with

```
R> alzheimer.ci$confint <- apply(alzheimer.ci$confint, 2,
+                                binomial()$linkinv)
R> plot(alzheimer.ci, main = "", xlim = c(0, 1))
```

see Figure 4.16. Using this graphical display of the results, it becomes evident that Alzheimer's disease is less frequent in men who smoke heavily compared to all other combinations of the two covariates. This result matches the findings from Salib and Hillier (1997). Note that these conclusions are drawn while controlling the familywise error rate in the strong sense.

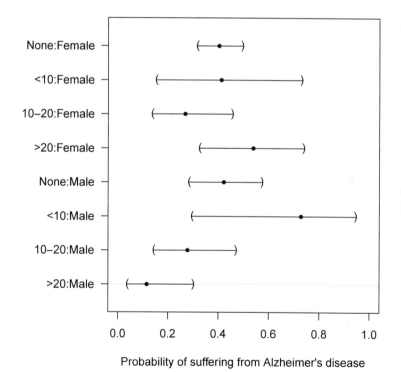

Figure 4.16   Simultaneous confidence intervals for the probability of suffering from Alzheimer's disease.

4.8 Multiple comparisons in survival models

The treatment of patients suffering from acute myeloid leukemia (AML) is determined by a tumor classification scheme which takes various cytogenetic aberration statuses into account. Bullinger, Döhner, Bair, Fröhlich, Schlenk, Tibshirani, Döhner, and Pollack (2004) investigated an extended tumor classification scheme incorporating molecular subgroups of the disease obtained by gene expression profiling. The analyses reported here are based on clinical data (thus omitting available gene expression data) published online at www.ncbi.nlm.nih.gov/geo, accession number GSE425. The overall survival time and censoring indicator as well as the clinical variables age, sex, lactic dehydrogenase level (LDH), white blood cell count (WBC), and treatment group are taken from Supplementary Table 1 in Bullinger et al. (2004). In addition, this table provides two molecular markers, the fmslike tyrosine kinase 3 (FLT3) and the mixed-lineage leukemia (MLL) gene, as well as cytogenetic information helpful in defining a risk score (low: karyotype t(8;21), t(15;17) and inv(16); intermediate: normal karyotype and t(9;11); and high: all other forms). One interesting question focuses on the usefulness of this risk score.

Using the survreg function from the **survival** package, we fit a Weibull survival model that includes all above mentioned covariates as well as their interactions with the patient's gender. We use the results from Chapter 3 to apply a suitable multiple comparison procedure, which accounts for the asymptotic correlations between the test statistics. We compare the three groups low, intermediate, and high using Tukey's all pairwise comparisons method described in Section 4.2. The output below indicates a difference when comparing high to both low and intermediate. The output also shows that low and intermediate are indistinguishable,

```
R> library("survival")
R> aml.surv <- survreg(Surv(time, event) ~ Sex +
+       Age + WBC + LDH + FLT3 + risk,
+       data = clinical)
R> summary(glht(aml.surv, linfct = mcp(risk = "Tukey")))

        Simultaneous Tests for General Linear Hypotheses

Multiple Comparisons of Means: Tukey Contrasts


Fit: survreg(formula = Surv(time, event) ~ Sex + Age + WBC +
   LDH + FLT3 + risk, data = clinical)


Linear Hypotheses:
                        Estimate Std. Error z value Pr(>|z|)
intermediate - high == 0   1.110      0.385    2.88   0.0108
low - high == 0            1.477      0.458    3.22   0.0036
low - intermediate == 0    0.367      0.430    0.85   0.6692
(Adjusted p values reported -- single-step method)
```

4.9 Multiple comparisons in mixed-effects models

In most parts of Germany, the natural or artificial regeneration of forests is difficult because of intensive animal browsing. Young trees suffer from browsing damage, mostly by roe and red deer. In order to estimate the browsing intensity for several tree species, the Bavarian State Ministry of Agriculture and Forestry conducts a survey every three years. Based on the estimated percentage of damaged trees, the ministry makes suggestions for implementing or modifying deer management programs. The survey takes place in all 756 game management districts in Bavaria. Here, we focus on the 2006 data of the game management district number 513 "Hegegemeinschaft Unterer Aischgrund",

```
R> data("trees513", package = "multcomp")
```

The data of 2700 trees include the species and a binary variable indicating whether or not the tree suffers from damage caused by deer browsing. Figure 4.17 displays the layout of the field experiment. A pre-specified, equally spaced grid was laid over the district. Within each of the resulting 36 rectangular areas, a 100m transect was identified on which 5 equidistant plots were determined (that is, a plot after every 25m). At each plot, 15 trees were observed, resulting in 75 trees for each area, or 2700 trees in total.

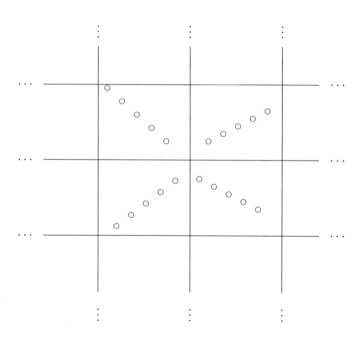

Figure 4.17   Layout of the trees513 field experiment. Each open dot denotes a plot with 15 trees. Further explanations are provided in the text.

We are interested in the probability estimates and the confidence intervals for each of six tree species under investigation. We fit a mixed-effects logistic regression model using the lmer function from the **lme4** package (Bates and Sarkar 2010). We exclude the intercept but include random effects accounting for the spatial variation of the trees. Thus, we have six fixed parameters, one for each of the six tree species, and $\mathbf{C} = \mathrm{diag}(6)$ is the matrix defining our experimental questions,

```
R> trees513.lme <- lmer(damage ~ species -1 + (1 | lattice/plot),
+                            data = trees513, family = binomial())
R> K <- diag(length(fixef(trees513.lme)))
```

We first compute simultaneous confidence intervals for the linear functions of interest and then transform these into the required probabilities,

```
R> trees513.ci <- confint(glht(trees513.lme, linfct = K))
R> prob <- binomial()$linkinv(trees513.ci$confint)
R> trees513.ci$confint <- 1 - prob
R> trees513.ci$confint[, 2:3] <- trees513.ci$confint[, 3:2]
```

The results are shown in Figure 4.18. Browsing is less frequent in hardwood. In particular, small oak trees are at high risk. As a consequence, the ministry has decided to increase the harvestry of roe deers in the following years. Relatively small sample sizes caused the large confidence intervals for ash, maple, elm and lime trees.

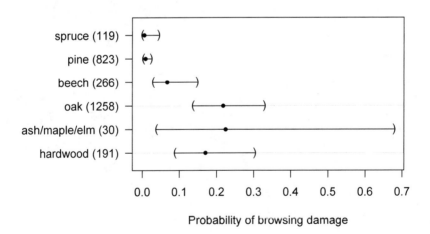

Figure 4.18 Probability of roe deer browsing damage for six tree species. Sample sizes are given in brackets.

CHAPTER 5

Further Topics

In this chapter we review a selection of multiple comparison problems, which do not quite fit into the framework of Chapters 3 and 4. The selection reflects a biased choice from a large number of possible topics and was partly driven by the availability of software implementations in R. In Section 5.1 we discuss the comparison of means with two-sample multivariate data using resampling-based methods. In Section 5.2 we review group sequential and adaptive designs, which allow for repeated significance testing while controlling the Type I error rate. Finally, in Section 5.3 we extend the ideas from Section 4.3 and describe a hybrid methodology combining multiple comparisons with modeling techniques for dose finding experiments. Because the individual sections in this chapter are not directly linked to previous parts of this book, separate notation is introduced where needed.

5.1 Resampling-based multiple comparison procedures

Resampling-based multiple comparison procedures have been investigated systematically since Westfall and Young (1993) and Troendle (1995); see also Dudoit and van der Laan (2008) for a description of such multiple comparison procedures relevant to genomics. In this section we discuss in detail the comparison of means with two-sample multivariate data using resampling-based methods. The general case of multi-sample multivariate data is not considered here and we refer to Westfall and Troendle (2008) for a recent discussion.

In Section 5.1.1, we describe the technical details underlying permutation-based multiple test procedures for two-sample multivariate data. To illustrate the methodology, we analyze two datasets in Section 5.1.2 using the **coin** package (Hothorn, Hornik, van de Wiel, and Zeileis 2010b), which allows us to use R for permutation multiple testing. In Section 5.1.3 we briefly review related bootstrap-based multiple test procedures.

5.1.1 Permutation methods

General considerations

With the closure principle from Section 2.2.3 in place, permutation-based multiple test procedures are often quite simple. All that is required is a permutation test for every intersection null hypothesis. Advantages of permutation tests are

(i) the resulting multiple test inference procedure is exact, despite non-normal characteristics of the data, and despite unknown covariance structures;

(ii) the resulting multiple comparison procedures incorporate correlations, like the max-t-based methods, to become less conservative than typical Bonferroni-based procedures;

(iii) in cases with sparse data, permutation-based methods offer quantum improvements over standard methods, in the sense that the effective number of tests m' can be much less than the actual number of tests m.

Coupled with (i) and (ii), the final point (iii) suggests a major benefit. Assume, for example, that $m = 30$ tests are performed for a specific analysis. Applying the simple-minded Bonferroni test leads to a critical value at level $0.05/30 = 0.0017$. But using permutation tests the effective number of tests can be substantially lower. If the data are sparse it might be as small as $m' = 4$ (or even smaller, as seen in the example from Table 5.1). This gives a Bonferroni critical value at level $0.05/4 = 0.0125$, thus leading to considerably higher power. A further benefit is that permutation-based methods use the correlation structure, so that the actual critical value will be higher still than the Bonferroni-based $0.05/4 = 0.0125$, as high as 0.05 itself (that is, no adjustment at all), depending on the nature of the dependence structure.

To understand the key concepts, it helps to go through an example, step-by-step. The dataset displayed in Table 5.1 is a mock-up adverse event (side effects) dataset from a safety analysis for a new drug, with three possible events E_1, E_2, and E_3. There are four total adverse events in the treatment group for E_1, and none in the control group. There is only one total adverse event observed for E_2 and E_3.

Group	E_1	E_2	E_3
Trt	1	1	1
Trt	1	0	0
Trt	1	0	0
Trt	1	0	0
Ctrl	0	0	0
Ctrl	0	0	0
Ctrl	0	0	0

Table 5.1   Mock-up dataset from a safety analysis for a new drug. The entry "1" denotes an observed adverse event; otherwise "0" is used.

Typically for two-sample binary data permutation tests, the test statistic is the total number of occurrences in the treatment group, and the one-sided p-value is the proportion of permutations yielding a total greater or equal to the observed total. This is known as Fisher's exact test. In the example dataset from Table 5.1, there are 7! possible permutations of the observations, but many of these are redundant. For example, the permutation that switches observations 1 and 2 (i.e., the first two rows), but leaves the remaining observations unchanged is redundant with the original dataset, since the same observations are in the treatment group as before, and the test statistic cannot change. There are $7!/(4!3!) = 35$ non-redundant permutations of the observations. For E_1, only one of these permutations yields 4 occurrences in the treated group, hence the Fisher exact upper-tailed p-value is $1/35 = 0.0286$. For E_2 and E_3, the single observed occurrence can take place in the treatment group for $4/7 = 0.5714$ of the permutations, hence the upper tailed p-values for E_2 and E_3 are 0.5714.

To implement the closed test procedure to judge the significance of the tests when the familywise error rate is controlled, we need to specify suitable tests for all intersection hypotheses. Figure 5.1 shows all the intersection hypotheses schematically. The null hypotheses are

$$H_I \colon F_I^T = F_I^C, \quad I \subseteq \{1, 2, 3\},$$

which states that the joint distributions F_I^T and F_I^C of the measurements in the set I are identical for treated and control groups, respectively. Each of these hypotheses can be tested "exactly" by

(i) selecting a statistic t_I to test H_I;

(ii) enumerating the permutations of the treatment/control labels, and finding the value of t_I^* for each permutation;

(iii) rejecting H_I at level α if the proportion of permutation samples yielding $t_I^* \geq t_I$ is less than or equal to α.

The reason that "exactly" is used in quotes is that the familywise error rate may be strictly less than α due to discreteness of the permutation distribution of t_I. However, the familywise error rate is guaranteed to be no more than α. Another reason for quotes around the term "exactly" is that with a large sample size, typically the permutation distribution must be randomly sampled rather than enumerated completely, and in such cases the method is not "exact", even though the simulation error can be reduced with sufficient sampling. With these caveats, the method controls the familywise error rate in the strong sense, with no approximation, provided that the true null state of nature is one of the states shown in the closure tree of Figure 5.1.

A comment is in order concerning the statement, "provided that the true null state of nature is one of the states shown in the closure tree." This statement is in fact an assumption needed for permutation tests based on the closure principle. It is possible, for example, that the marginal distributions are equal but the joint distributions are not, and the methods discussed in this chapter do not control the familywise error rate under this scenario. On the other hand, if the joint distributions are not equal for some subsets, then it is a fact that the treatment differs from the control, so the determination of some significant difference in that case is correct, even though some spe-

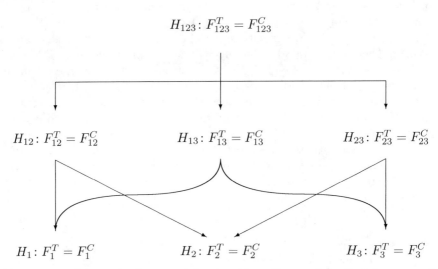

Figure 5.1   Schematic diagram of the closed hypotheses set for the adverse event data.

cific determinations regarding marginal significances might be erroneous. An example where this assumption fails is where the treatment has no effect on the marginal rates of occurrences of adverse events E_1 and E_2, but does affect the joint distribution of the occurrences. This assumption is called the *joint exchangeability assumption* by Westfall and Troendle (2008).

In the following we continue the discussion in terms of min-p tests instead of the max-t tests introduced in Equation (2.1) and used throughout this book. The results are equivalent in standard parametric applications when one takes $t_i = F_i^{-1}(1 - p_i)$, where F_i denotes the distribution of the test statistic t_i. The explanation that follows differs slightly in that permutation-based p-values are used.

In the adverse events example above, the hypothesis $H_{123}\colon F_{123}^T = F_{123}^C$ is tested using the min-p statistic $t_{123} = \min\{p_1, p_2, p_3\}$. Note that for each permutation of the dataset, different p-values are obtained; call p_i^* the p-value for a random permutation. The global p-value for testing H_{123} is then the proportion of the $7!/(4!3!) = 35$ permutations of the dataset (where the rows are kept intact and only the treatment/control labels are permuted) for which $\min\{p_1^*, p_2^*, p_3^*\}$ is less than or equal to $\min\{p_1, p_2, p_3\}$. In this example $\min\{p_1, p_2, p_3\} = \min\{0.0286, 0.5714, 0.5714\} = 0.0286$.

Here is where the advantage of permutation testing for sparse data becomes evident. Notice that the possible p-values p_1^* for E_1 are either 1.0000, 0.8857, 0.3714, or 0.0286, corresponding to 1, 2, 3, or 4 occurrences in the treatment group, respectively. For E_2 and E_3, the possible p_i^* are either 1.0000 or 0.5714, corresponding to 0 or 1 occurrences in the treatment group, respectively. Thus, it is impossible for p_i^*, $i = 2, 3$, to be smaller than 0.0286, hence the p-value for H_{123}, $p_{123} = \mathbb{P}(\min \{p_1^*, p_2^*, p_3^*\} \leq 0.0286) = \mathbb{P}(p_1^* \leq 0.0286) = 0.0286$. Similarly, $p_{12} = 0.0286$, $p_{13} = 0.0286$, and of course $p_1 = 0.0286$. Hence, the exact multiplicity-adjusted p-value for testing E_1 is identical to the unadjusted p-value, due to the sparseness of the data in the E_2 and E_3 variables.

Even when the data are not sparse, there are still benefits from permutation tests. To illustrate, consider the 2×2 contingency tables in Table 5.2 that show the pattern of occurrences for two variables E_1 and E_2. The Fisher exact upper-tailed p-value for E_1 is $p_1 = 0.0261$, and that for E_2 is $p_2 = 0.0790$. The standard Holm and Hochberg methods fail to find significances at level $\alpha = 0.05$, with adjusted p-values $q_1 = 0.0523$ and $q_2 = 0.0790$.

	E_1			E_2		
	Event	Non-Event	Total	Event	Non-Event	Total
Trt	7	43	50	8	43	51
Ctrl	1	51	52	3	52	55
Total	8	94	102	11	95	106

Table 5.2 Two contingency tables for two types of adverse events E_1 (left) and E_2 (right). Differing sample sizes are due to missing values.

However, using permutation tests within the closure paradigm we obtain $q_1 \leq 0.0451$ and $q_2 = 0.0790$. To see why, examine the graphs in Figure 5.2 of the distribution of the possible number of treatment occurrences of E_1 and E_2, based on the hypergeometric distributions $H(x, 50, 8, 102)$ and $H(x, 51, 11, 106)$ when the total number of events is 8 and 11, respectively. From these distributions, the tail probabilities give the possible Fisher upper-tailed p-values for each of the two tests; see Table 5.3. The p-value for H_{12} is $\mathbb{P}(\min \{p_1^*, p_2^*\} \leq 0.0261)$. But

$$
\begin{aligned}
\mathbb{P}(\min\{p_1^*, p_2^*\} \leq 0.0261) &\leq \mathbb{P}(p_1^* \leq 0.0261) + \mathbb{P}(p_2^* \leq 0.0261) \\
&= 0.0261 + 0.0190 \\
&= 0.0451,
\end{aligned}
$$

where, from Table 5.2, 0.0190 is the probability that p_2^* is less than or equal to 0.0261, and where the inequality in the first line follows from the Bonferroni inequality (2.3). Thus, the adjusted p-value for H_1 is $\max \{\mathbb{P}(\min\{p_1^*, p_2^*\} \leq 0.0261), \mathbb{P}(p_1^* \leq 0.0261)\} \leq 0.0451$. Permutation tests take advantage of discreteness of the permutation distributions to reduce the p-values and hence improve power.

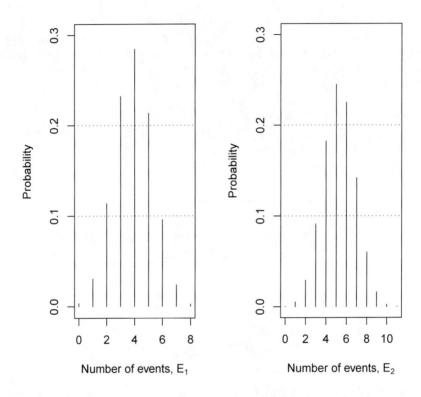

Figure 5.2   Histograms of the hypergeometric distributions $H(x, 50, 8, 102)$ and
$H(x, 51, 11, 106)$ for the adverse event data in Table 5.2.

The permutation multiple test algorithm

Recently, there is great interest in high-dimensional multiple testing, where
the number of variables far exceeds the sample size. Gene expression is a
prototype application, but the applications are much broader. Permutation-
based methods have become popular for "-omics" because they (i) require fewer
assumptions (such as normality) about the data-generating process, thereby
yielding procedures that are more robust, and (ii) utilize data-based distributional characteristics, such as discreteness and correlation structure, to make
tests more powerful.

It might seem from Figure 5.1, which shows the closure tree for three variables, that the closure method would become difficult to compute for large m,
since the number of nodes in the tree is in general $2^m - 1$. However, it turns
out that the method scales up, computationally, to very large m, provided one

E_1		E_2	
Trt Events	p-value	Trt Events	p-value
0	1.00	0	1.00
1	0.9966	1	0.9996
2	0.9661	2	0.9942
3	0.8523	3	0.9650
4	0.6201	4	0.8738
5	0.3357	5	0.6914
6	0.1222	6	0.4465
7	0.0261	7	0.2211
8	0.0025	8	0.0790
-		9	0.0190
-		10	0.0027
-		11	0.0002

Table 5.3   Upper-tailed p-values for the adverse event data in Table 5.2.

can make two simplifying assumptions that drastically reduce the computing burden from $\mathcal{O}(2^m)$ to $\mathcal{O}(m)$. These concepts are described here briefly, but see Westfall and Troendle (2008) for further details.

The first simplifying assumption, one made throughout this book, is that each intersection hypothesis H_I is tested using either a min-p statistic $\min_{i \in I} p_i$ or a max-t statistic $\max_{i \in I} t_i$; see also Equation (2.1). The second is the "subset pivotality" assumption coined by Westfall and Young (1993), which states that the distribution of $\max_{i \in I} t_i$ is identical under H_I and $H = H_M$ for all $I \subseteq M = \{1, \ldots, m\}$. If the first assumption is met, one need only test m hypotheses corresponding to the ordered t_i rather than all $2^m - 1$ intersections. In addition, if the second assumption is met, permutation resampling can be done simultaneously for all m tests using the global null hypothesis H, rather than perform permutation resampling separately for each of the m intersection hypotheses corresponding to the ordered test statistics. The subset pivotality assumption fails notably when testing pairwise comparisons of distributions in the case of multiple treatment groups. In this case, use of the global permutation distribution, which states exhangeability among all treatment groups, cannot be used to test for exchangeability among two of the treatment groups, as differences in variability among the treatment groups can cause bias in the statistical tests. There are several ways that one might perform permutation tests correctly in this case; see Petrondas and Gabriel (1983) for one solution.

The subset pivotality assumption is mainly used to simplify computations in the closed test algorithm. Along with the use of max-t statistics, it provides a shortcut procedure that allows the researcher to test the m hypotheses corresponding to the ordered p-values, rather than all $2^m - 1$ intersection hypotheses. If it is possible to test all $2^m - 1$ hypotheses using valid permutation tests, then subset pivotality is not needed for multiple testing using permutation tests. Note that shortcut procedures can also be derived under other assumptions than subset pivotality; see Calian, Li, and Hsu (2008) for a recent discussion.

Suppose the observed test statistics are $t_1^{\text{obs}} \geq \ldots \geq t_m^{\text{obs}}$, corresponding to hypotheses $H_1, \ldots, H_m$, and that larger t_i^{obs} suggest alternative hypotheses. Suppose a p-value for testing H_I using the statistic $\max_{i \in I} t_i$ is available. Then,

$$p_I = P\left(\max_{i \in I} t_i \geq \max_{i \in I} t_i^{\text{obs}} \,\middle|\, H_I \right),$$

and H_I is rejected at unadjusted level α if $p_I \leq \alpha$. The closure method along with the assumptions of use of max-t tests and of subset pivotality give the following algorithm for rejecting sequentially the ordered hypotheses $H_1, H_2, \ldots$

Step 1: By closure,

$$\text{reject } H_1 \text{ if } \max_{I:\, I \supseteq \{1\}} P\left(\max_{i \in I} t_i \geq \max_{i \in I} t_i^{\text{obs}} \,\middle|\, H_I \right) \leq \alpha.$$

But if $I \supseteq \{1\}$, then $\max_{i \in I} t_i^{\text{obs}} = t_1^{\text{obs}}$ and the rule is

$$\text{reject } H_1 \text{ if } \max_{I:\, I \supseteq \{1\}} P\left(\max_{i \in I} t_i \geq t_1^{\text{obs}} \,\middle|\, H_I \right) \leq \alpha.$$

Using subset pivotality, the rule becomes

$$\text{reject } H_1 \text{ if } \max_{I:\, I \supseteq \{1\}} P\left(\max_{i \in I} t_i \geq t_1^{\text{obs}} \,\middle|\, H \right) \leq \alpha.$$

Use of the max-t statistic implies

$$P\left(\max_{i \in I} t_i \geq t_1^{\text{obs}} \,\middle|\, H \right) \leq P\left(\max_{i \in J} t_i \geq t_1^{\text{obs}} \,\middle|\, H \right) \text{ for } I \subseteq J.$$

Hence, by subset pivotality and by use of the max-t statistic, the rule by which we reject H_1 simplifies to

$$\text{reject } H_1 \text{ if } P\left(\max_{i \in M} t_i \geq t_1^{\text{obs}} \,\middle|\, H \right) \leq \alpha.$$

Step 2: Again by closure and subset pivotality,

$$\text{reject } H_2 \text{ if } \max_{I:\, I \supseteq \{2\}} P\left(\max_{i \in I} t_i \geq \max_{i \in I} t_i^{\text{obs}} \,\middle|\, H \right) \leq \alpha.$$

If $I \supseteq \{1\}$, then $\max_{i \in I} t_i^{\text{obs}} = t_1^{\text{obs}}$; else $\max_{i \in I} t_i^{\text{obs}} = t_2^{\text{obs}}$. Partitioning the set $\{I: I \supseteq \{2\}\}$ into two sets,

$$S_1 = \{I: I \supseteq \{1,2\}\} \text{ and } S_2 = \{I: I \supseteq \{2\}, I \not\supseteq \{1\}\},$$

we require

$$P\left(\max_{i \in I} t_i \geq t_1^{\text{obs}} \,\middle|\, H \right) \leq \alpha \text{ for all } I \in S_1$$

and

$$P\left(\max_{i\in I} t_i \geq t_2^{\mathrm{obs}}\,\Big|\,H\right) \leq \alpha \text{ for all } I \in S_2.$$

Since we are using the max-t statistic, these conditions allow us to reject H_2 if

$$P\left(\max_{i\in M} t_i \geq t_1^{\mathrm{obs}}\,\Big|\,H\right) \leq \alpha$$

and

$$P\left(\max_{i\in\{2,\ldots,m\}} t_i \geq t_2^{\mathrm{obs}}\,\Big|\,H\right) \leq \alpha.$$

$\vdots$

Step j: Continuing in this fashion, we reject H_j if

$$P\left(\max_{i\in M} t_i \geq t_1^{\mathrm{obs}}\,\Big|\,H\right) \leq \alpha,$$

and

$$P\left(\max_{i\in\{2,\ldots,m\}} t_i \geq t_2^{\mathrm{obs}}\,\Big|\,H\right) \leq \alpha,$$

$$\cdots,$$

and

$$P\left(\max_{i\in\{j,\ldots,m\}} t_i \geq t_j^{\mathrm{obs}}\,\Big|\,H\right) \leq \alpha.$$

$\vdots$

Note that at step j in the algorithm we can equivalently reject H_j, if $\max_{i\leq j} p_{i\ldots m} \leq \alpha$. Hence, the rejection rule reduces to

$$\text{reject } H_j \text{ if } q_j \leq \alpha,$$

where $q_j = \max_{i\leq j} p_{i\ldots m}$ denotes the adjusted p-value.

One need not use resampling at all to apply the algorithm above. It only becomes a resampling-based procedure if one uses resampling to obtain the probabilities $P\left(\max_{i\in\{j,\ldots,m\}} t_i \geq t_j^{\mathrm{obs}}\,\big|\,H\right)$. In Section 4.1.2 we presented a similar algorithm, where the necessary probabilities are computed from the multivariate normal or t distribution.

In addition to subset pivotality and use of max-t statistics, we also assumed that there are no logical constraints among the hypotheses (recall Section 2.1.2 for the definition of the restricted combination property). This assumption is needed to assert that the algorithm is identical to closed testing using max-t statistics. If there are logical constraints, power can be improved by restricting attention only to admissible subsets I. In this case, shortcut procedures are more difficult to derive; see Brannath and Bretz (2010) for details. The algorithm above can still be used for logically constrained hypotheses, though, despite not being fully closed, as it provides a conservative procedure relative to the fully closed algorithm.

Comments on subset pivotality

Subset pivotality is most problematic in cases where there are multiple (i.e., $m > 2$) groups, especially when there are drastic differences in variability between the groups. Specifically, suppose the data are univariate, in three groups $i = 1, 2, 3$. Assume further that we are interested in the pairwise equality hypotheses $H_{ij} \colon F_i = F_j$, tested using permutation distributions of test statistics $t_{ij} = \bar{x}_i - \bar{x}_j$. Subset pivotality requires, for example, that the permutation distribution of $\bar{x}_1 - \bar{x}_2$ is identical, no matter whether one permutes the data between the groups 1 and 2 alone, excluding group 3, or by permuting the entire dataset. In the latter case, data from all three groups is involved, in the former case only data from groups 1 and 2 is involved. When data from group 3 differ dramatically, particularly in the variance, the global permutation distribution can be far different from the local distribution, and provide very bad results. The problem is nearly identical to the use of a pooled variance in linear model contrasts when the variances are quite different.

An example similar to one found in Westfall et al. (1999) illustrates the problem with count data. Suppose there are four treatment groups A, B, C, and D with the outcomes summarized in Table 5.4. The goal is to compare the three treatment groups B, C, and D with A, using permutation tests. The unadjusted upper-tailed Fisher exact p-values are $p_{BA} = 0.9041$, $p_{CA} = 0.0297$, and $p_{DA} = 0.1811$. If one uses the algorithm above, blindly, without considering the subset pivotality assumption, then the adjusted p-value for comparing C with A would be $q_{CA} = P(\min_i p_i \leq 0.0297 | H_{ABCD}) = 0.0049$, which is smaller than the unadjusted p-value. The problem is caused by the large amount of data in the B group with small variance; pooling this data with all other groups and permuting similarly drives down the variability, inappropriately, for the individual comparisons.

Group	Events	Sample Size
A	1	50
B	5	500
C	7	50
D	4	50

Table 5.4 Mock-up dataset with four treatment groups.

There are various fixes to the problem. One is to fit a binomial model allowing different variances for the groups, and proceeding with the multiple comparisons in approximate (asymptotic) fashion as described in Section 3.2. If exact inference is desired, it appears necessary to use the full closure. For example, to compare C with A, one needs exact p-values for H_{AC}, which is $p_{AC} = 0.0297$, as well as the intersection hypotheses H_{ABC}, H_{ACD}, and H_{ABCD}. The p-value for H_{ABCD} is shown above as $p_{ABCD} = 0.0049$. Deleting group B and D successively and recomputing, the remaining intersection p-values are $p_{\text{ACD}} = 0.0296$ and $p_{\text{ABC}} = 0.0012$. Hence, the correct, exact adjusted p-value is $q_{\text{CA}} = \max\{0.0297, 0.0296, 0.0012, 0.0049\} = 0.0297$. Once again, we see the fortunate case where the adjusted and unadjusted p-values do not differ, when exact permutation-based tests are used.

5.1.2 Using R for permutation multiple testing

R software for resampling-based multiple testing includes the **multtest** package (Pollard, Gilbert, Ge, Taylor, and Dudoit 2010); see Dudoit and van der Laan (2008) for mathematical details. Here, we analyze adverse event and multiple endpoint data with the **coin** package in R, which uses slightly different test statistics than disucussed in Section 5.1.1. Suppose that we are given observations $(\mathbf{y}_i, \mathbf{x}_i)$, where $\mathbf{y}_i$ denotes the individiual, possibly multivariate outcome and $\mathbf{x}_i$ denotes a binary treatment indicator, $i = 1, \ldots, n$. The multivariate linear test statistic

$$\mathbf{t} = \text{vec}\left(\sum_{i=1}^{n} I(\mathbf{x}_i = 1)\mathbf{y}_i^{\top}\right)$$

is a vector containing the sum over all observations within each treatment group. Strasser and Weber (1999) derived the conditional expectation $\boldsymbol{\mu}$ and covariance matrix $\boldsymbol{\Sigma}$ under the null hypothesis of independence between $\mathbf{y}$ and $\mathbf{x}$; see also Hothorn et al. (2006). Thus, we can use the standardized test statistic

$$\frac{\mathbf{t} - \boldsymbol{\mu}}{\text{diag}(\boldsymbol{\Sigma})^{1/2}}$$

and therefore obtain one statistic for each of the multiple outcome variables in $\mathbf{y}_i$. For binary responses, this corresponds (up to a factor $(n-1)/n$) to the root of the χ^2 test statistic in a two-by-two contingency table. For continuous responses, this is roughly equivalent to a t statistic.

Adverse events data

Testing adverse events in clinical trials is a common application. The dataset provided by Westfall et al. (1999, p. 242) contains binary indicators of 28 adverse events, denoted as E_1 through E_{28}. In R, we can set up a formula with the adverse event data on the left hand side and the treatment indicator on the right hand side:

```
R> data("adevent", package = "multcomp")
R> library("coin")
R> fm <- as.formula(paste(
+       paste("E", 1:28, sep = "", collapse = "+"),
+       "~ group"))
R> fm
```

```
E1 + E2 + E3 + E4 + E5 + E6 + E7 + E8 + E9 + E10 + E11 + E12 +
    E13 + E14 + E15 + E16 + E17 + E18 + E19 + E20 + E21 + E22 +
    E23 + E24 + E25 + E26 + E27 + E28 ~ group
```

The permutation distribution of the data (for 10,000 random permutations) is evaluated using the `independence_test` function. Its output provides the necessary information to inspect the standardized statistics and the corresponding adjusted p-values:

```
R> it <- independence_test(fm, data = adevent,
+       distribution = approximate(B = 10000))
R> statistic(it, "standardized")

  E1.no event E2.no event E3.no event E4.no event E5.no event
A        3.31      -0.256       0.311      -0.342        1.16
  E6.no event E7.no event E8.no event E9.no event E10.no event
A        2.02      -0.453        2.26       -1.01        1.42
  E11.no event E12.no event E13.no event E14.no event
A          -1        -1.42          -1        -1.42
  E15.no event E16.no event E17.no event E18.no event
A        1.42            0          -1          -1
  E19.no event E20.no event E21.no event E22.no event
A       -1.42            1           0          -1
  E23.no event E24.no event E25.no event E26.no event
A           1           -1          -1          -1
  E27.no event E28.no event
A          -1        0.318
```

```
R> pvalue(it, method = "single-step")

  E1.no event E2.no event E3.no event E4.no event E5.no event
A       0.003            1            1            1            1
  E6.no event E7.no event E8.no event E9.no event E10.no event
A       0.276            1        0.113            1        0.708
  E11.no event E12.no event E13.no event E14.no event
A           1        0.708            1        0.708
  E15.no event E16.no event E17.no event E18.no event
A       0.708            1            1            1
  E19.no event E20.no event E21.no event E22.no event
A       0.708            1            1            1
  E23.no event E24.no event E25.no event E26.no event
A           1            1            1            1
  E27.no event E28.no event
A           1            1
```

The null hypothesis of equal distribution of the events in both treatment arms can be rejected only for E_1. The above analysis is the single-step test procedure implemented in the **coin** package. Step-down testing can be accomplished by successively excluding adverse events according to the size of the test statistics, and repeating the analysis.

Analysis of multiple endpoints

A dataset described in Westfall, Krishen, and Young (1998) contains measurements of patients in treatment (active drug) and control (placebo) groups, with four outcome variables (i.e., endpoints) labeled E_1, E_2, E_3, and E_4. Table 5.5 displays the summary statistics.

	Sample Size	Mean	Standard deviation
Control			
E_1	54	2.4444	4.3683
E_2	54	3.2222	1.4623
E_3	54	2.7778	1.6673
E_4	54	3.2593	1.6390
Treatment			
E_1	57	0.9298	1.3740
E_2	57	2.5439	1.3372
E_3	57	2.4035	1.3740
E_4	57	2.5088	1.6810

Table 5.5 Summary results of a study with two treatments and four outcome variables.

Using the **coin** package, we again apply the `independence_test` function to investigate deviations from the null hypotheses that each response variables' distribution is the same in both arms. Here, the permutation distribution of all four test statistics are approximated by 50.000 random permutations of the data:

```
R> data("mtept", package = "multcomp")
R> it <- independence_test(E1 + E2 + E3 + E4 ~ treatment,
+      data = mtept, distribution = approximate(B = 50000))
R> statistic(it, "standardized")

        E1    E2    E3    E4
Drug -2.49 -2.43 -1.29 2.33

R> pvalue(it, method = "single-step")

        E1      E2     E3     E4
Drug 0.0343 0.0409 0.489 0.0525
```

Differences between treatment groups can be postulated for all except the third outcome variable.

5.1.3 Bootstrap testing – Brief overview

Bootstrap testing is related to permutation testing. The simplest comparison is that bootstrap sampling is done with replacement, while permutation sampling is done without replacement, but there is more to it than that. Briefly, one advantage of bootstrap testing is that it can be performed using a wider class of models, for example, those with covariates, while permutation testing applies to a more rigid class of models. A disadvantage of bootstrap testing is that it is always inexact and approximate, especially for a popular separate sample type of bootstrap. Troendle, Korn, and McShane (2004) demonstrated spectacular failure of the separate sample bootstrap for genomics applications compared to the more reasonable approximations of the pooled bootstrap and the exactness of the permutational approach. For typical linear models applications involving pairwise comparisons, the parametric approximation and bootstrap approximation give reasonably similar results, despite nonnormality (Bretz and Hothorn 2003). A case where bootstrapping is necessary for multiple comparisons, works well, and where other methods are not available is given by Westfall and Young (1993, Section 2.5.1).

5.2 Methods for group sequential and adaptive designs

In standard experiments, the sample size is fixed and calculated based on the assumed effect sizes, variability, etc. to achieve a designated power level while controlling the Type I error rate. In sequential sampling schemes, the sample size is not fixed, but a random variable. Interim analyses are performed during an ongoing experiment to make conclusions before the end of the experiment or allow one to adjust for incorrect assumptions at the design stage. For example, when interim results suggest a change in sample sizes for the subsequent stages, sample size reestimation methods become an important tool (Chuang-Stein, Anderson, Gallo, and Collins 2006). However, repeatedly looking at the data with the possibility for interim decision making may inflate the overall Type I error rate and appropriate analysis methods are required to guarantee its strong control at a pre-specified significance level α.

Group sequential and adaptive designs are particularly widely applied in clinical trials because of ethical and financial reasons. Patients should not be treated with inefficacious treatments and interim analyses offer the possibility to stop a trial early for futility (i.e., lack of efficacy). On the other hand, efficacious and safe treatments should be released quickly to the market so that patients in need can benefit from the potentially ground-breaking therapy. In Section 5.2.1 we describe the basic theory of group sequential designs and illustrate the methodology with a numerical example using the **gsDesign** package in R (Anderson 2010). In Section 5.2.2 we briefly review adaptive designs and describe the **asd** package (Parsons 2010).

5.2.1 Group sequential designs

In this section we focus on group sequential designs, which have received much attention since Pocock (1977) and O'Brien and Fleming (1979). It is not the aim of this section to develop the theory in detail. Instead, we refer to the books by Jennison and Turnbull (2000) and Proschan, Lan, and Wittes (2006) for a complete mathematical treatise of this subject. For details on **gsDesign** we refer to the manual accompanying the package (Anderson 2010).

Basic theory

Consider normally distributed responses with unknown mean θ and known variance σ^2. Assume that we are interested in testing the null hypothesis $H : \theta = \theta_0$ (the one-sided case is treated similarly). Assume further that there is interest in stopping the trial early either for success (reject the null hypothesis H) or for futility (retain H). In group sequential designs, inspections are made after groups of observations. Assume a maximum number k of inspections for some positive integer k. The first $k - 1$ analyses are referred to as interim analyses, while the k-th analysis is referred to as the final analysis.

Let n_i, $i = 1, \ldots, k$, denote the sample sizes in the k sequences of observations. Further, let $\bar{x}_i$ denote the mean value at stage i. For $i = 1, \ldots, k$ consider the overall standardized test statistics

$$z_i^* = \frac{\sum_{j=1}^{i} \sqrt{n_j} z_j}{\sqrt{\sum_{j=1}^{i} n_j}},$$

where $z_i = \sqrt{n_i}(\bar{x}_i - \theta_0)/\sigma$ denotes the test statistic from the ith stage of the trial. The test statistics $z_1^*, \ldots, z_k^*$ are jointly multivariate normally distributed with means

$$\eta_i = \mathbb{E}(z_i^*) = \frac{\theta - \theta_0}{\sigma} \sqrt{\sum_{j=1}^{i} n_j}$$

and covariances

$$\mathbb{V}(t_i, t_{i'}) = \sqrt{\frac{t_i}{t_{i'}}},$$

where $i \leq i'$ and $t_i = \sum_{j=1}^{i} n_j / \sum_{j=1}^{k} n_j$ denotes the information fraction at stage i. As shown in Jennison and Turnbull (2000), this set-up is asymptotically valid in many practically relevant situations, including two-armed trials with normal, binary or time-to-event outcomes; see also Wassmer (1999) and Wassmer (2009).

A group sequential design consists of specifying the continuation regions C_i, $i = 1, \ldots, k - 1$, at the interim analyses and the acceptance region C_k at the final analysis. If at any interim analysis $z_i^* \notin C_i$, the trial stops and the null hypothesis H is rejected. Otherwise, the trial is continued as long as $z_i^* \in C_i$. If the trial continues until the final analysis and $z_i^* \in C_k$, the null hypothesis H is retained. That is, in this simplest case, the rejection region is the complement of the continuation region C_i, $i = 1, \ldots, k - 1$, and no other stopping rule is considered. Accordingly, any group sequential design needs to satisfy

$$\mathbb{P}_H \left(\bigcap_{i=1}^{k} \{z_i^* \in C_i\} \right) = 1 - \alpha.$$

The crossing boundaries defining the decision regions C_i can be computed efficiently by accounting for the special structure of the covariance matrix described above (Armitage, McPherson, and Rowe 1969). Once a group sequential design has been defined, the average sample size ASN is readily given by

$$\text{ASN} = n_1 + \sum_{i=2}^{k} n_i \mathbb{P}_{\boldsymbol{\eta}} \left(\bigcap_{j=1}^{i-1} \{z_i^* \in C_j\} \right),$$

where $\boldsymbol{\eta} = (\eta_1, \ldots, \eta_k)$ and η_i is defined above. As seen from the example further below, the average sample size can be used to assees the efficiency of group sequential designs as compared to fixed designs without interim analyses.

Many choices of C_i lead to valid group sequential designs, thus allowing the investigator to fine tune the trial design according to the study objectives. A common choice of group sequential designs is the Δ-class of boundaries introduced by Wang and Tsiatis (1987). They introduced a one-parameter class of symmetric boundaries, which in case of two-sided testing and equally spaced interim analyses are given by

$$C_i = (-u_i; u_i), \quad u_i = c(k, \alpha, \Delta) i^{\Delta - 0.5},$$

where the constant $c(k, \alpha, \Delta)$ is chosen appropriately to control the Type I error rate. Note that for $\Delta = 0.5$ the boundary values are all equal and thus lead to the well-known design of Pocock (1977). The value $\Delta = 0$ generates the design of O'Brien and Fleming (1979) as special case. Figure 5.3 displays the upper rejection boundaries from Wang and Tsiatis (1987) for $\Delta = 0, 0.25, 0.5$ in a group sequential trial with $k = 4$ analyses and $\alpha = 0.025$ (one-sided test problem).

The error spending function method proposed by Lan and DeMets (1983) is an alternative approach to define a group sequential design. The idea is to specify the cumulative Type I error rate $\alpha^*(t_i)$ spent up to the i-th interim analysis and derive the critical values based on these values. The function $\alpha^*(t_i)$ must be specified in advance and is assumed to be non-decreasing with $\alpha^*(0) = 0$ and $\alpha^*(1) = \alpha$. The time points t_i do not need to be pre-specified before the actual course of the trial. Consequently, the number of observations at the i-th analysis and the maximum number k of analyses are flexible, although their determination must be independent of any emerging data. In the two-sided case, the critical value for the first analysis is given by $u_1 = \Phi^{-1}(1 - \alpha^*(t_1)/2)$, where Φ denotes the cumulative distribution function of the standard normal distribution. The remaining critical values

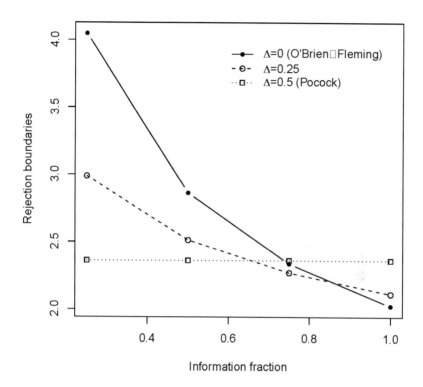

Figure 5.3 Several examples of rejection boundaries from Wang and Tsiatis (1987). Here, $\Delta = 0$ generates an O'Brien-Fleming design, while $\Delta = 0.5$ produces a Pocock design.

$u_2, \ldots, u_k$ are computed successively through

$$\mathbb{P}_H\left(\bigcap_{j=1}^{i-1}\{|z_j^*| < u_j\} \cap \{|z_i^*| \geq u_i\}\right) = \alpha^*(t_i) - \alpha^*(t_{i-1}).$$

The one-sided case is treated analogously.

Several choices for the form of the error spending function $\alpha^*(t_i)$ were proposed. The choices

$$\alpha^*(t_i) = \alpha \ln\left(1 + (e-1)t_i\right)$$

and

$$\alpha^*(t_i) = \begin{cases} 2\left(1 - \Phi\left(\frac{u_{1-\alpha/2}}{\sqrt{t_i}}\right)\right) & \text{(one-sided case)} \\ 4\left(1 - \Phi\left(\frac{u_{1-\alpha/4}}{\sqrt{t_i}}\right)\right) & \text{(two-sided case)} \end{cases}$$

approximate the group sequential boundaries from Pocock (1977) and O'Brien
and Fleming (1979), respectively, where $u_{1-p} = \Phi^{-1}(1-p)$. Likewise, Hwang,
Shih, and DeCani (1990) introduced the one-parameter family

$$\alpha^*(\gamma, t_i) = \begin{cases} \alpha \frac{1-\exp(-\gamma t_i)}{1-\exp(-\gamma)} & \text{for } \gamma \neq 0 \\ \alpha t_i & \text{for } \gamma = 0 \end{cases}$$

and showed that its use yields approximately optimal plans similar to the Δ-
class of Wang and Tsiatis (1987). A value of $\gamma = -4$ is used to approximate an
O'Brien-Fleming design, while a value of $\gamma = 1$ approximates a Pocock design
well. Figure 5.4 displays the error spending functions from Hwang et al. (1990)
for $\gamma = -4, -2, 1$.

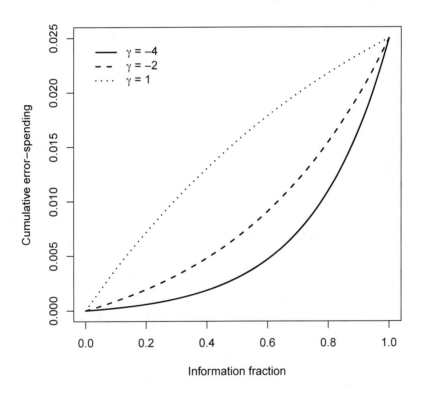

Figure 5.4   Several examples of error spending functions from Hwang et al. (1990)
for $\alpha = 0.025$. Here, $\gamma = -4$ approximates an O'Brien-Fleming design,
while $\gamma = 1$ approximates a Pocock design.

An example

In this section we use a numerical example to illustrate the above methodology with the **gsDesign** package, which supports the design of group sequential trials in R. Assume that we plan a one-sided group sequential design with 90% power to detect a standardized treatment effect size of $\theta_0 = 0.15$ to compare patients under treatment (active drug) and control (placebo). In the following, we show details for an O'Brien-Fleming design, which employs more stringent boundaries at early interim analyses than later. We plan for $k = 4$ equally spaced analyses and $\alpha = 0.025$, although the concepts below also apply to other design options.

The gsDesign function from the **gsDesign** package provides sample size and boundaries for a group sequential design based on treatment effects, spending functions for boundary crossing probabilities, and relative timing of each analysis. According to the trial specifications above, the call

```
R> library("gsDesign")
R> gsd.OF <- gsDesign(k = 4, test.type = 1, sfu = "OF",
+                     alpha = 0.025, beta = 0.1, timing = 1,
+                     delta = 0.15)
```

provides the relevant information. In this call, `test.type = 1` gives a one-sided test problem, `timing = 1` produces equally spaced analyses and `sfu` defines the error spending function (that is, O'Brien-Fleming in our example). All of the spending functions described in Section 5.2.1 as well as many other functions are implemented in the **gsDesign** package. Finally, `delta` defines the standardized treatment effect size for which the design is powered. Because of a different standardization used by the gsDesign function, `delta` has to be set as $\theta_0/2 = 0.15$; see Anderson (2010) for details.

The next line prints a summary of gsd.OF using the **print** method associated with **gsDesign** objects,

```
R> gsd.OF
```

```
One-sided group sequential design with
90 % power and 2.5 % Type I Error.

  Analysis  N    Z    Nominal p  Spend
         1 120 4.05    0.0000 0.0000
         2 239 2.86    0.0021 0.0021
         3 359 2.34    0.0097 0.0083
         4 478 2.02    0.0215 0.0145
     Total                    0.0250
++ alpha spending:
 O'Brien-Fleming boundary

Boundary crossing probabilities and expected sample size
assume any cross stops the trial

Upper boundary (power or Type I Error)
```

```
      Analysis
 Theta     1       2        3        4  Total  E{N}
  0.00 0.000  0.0021  0.0083  0.0145  0.025   476
  0.15 0.008  0.2850  0.4031  0.2040  0.900   358
```

The upper table of the output contains for each of the $k = 4$ analyses the cumulative total sample size N, the (upper) rejection bound Z, the one-sided significance level Nominal p, and the error spent. In this example, roughly 120 patients are required at each of the four stages to ensure a power of 90% (recall that we asked for equally spaced interim analyses). This leads to a maximum of 478 patients that are required for this design. For comparison, the sample size in a fixed design (without interim analyses) is 467. Thus, the maximum sample size in the group sequential design is 1.02 times the sample size in a fixed-sample design. This inflation factor relates the sample size of a group sequential design to its corresponding fixed design and can be obtained with gsDesign by setting delta = 0:

```
R> gsd.OF2 <- gsDesign(k = 4, test.type = 1,
+        sfu = "OF", alpha = 0.025, beta = 0.1, timing = 1,
+        delta = 0)
R> gsd.OF2$n.I[4]
```

```
[1] 1.02
```

Figure 5.5 plots the upper stopping boundaries

```
[1] 4.05 2.86 2.34 2.02
```

against the cumulative sample sizes

```
[1] 119 239 358 477
```

for the selected O'Brien-Fleming design. The area above the displayed curve is the rejection region: Whenever the test statistic crosses the boundary at an interim analysis, one can reject the null hypothesis and stop the trial early for success. Figure 5.5 was produced using the plot method associated with the gsDesign function; see below for further plotting capabilities.

The inflation factor introduced above is independent of the standardized effect size, the test and the outcome of interest and serves as basis for sample size calculations in group sequential designs. However, it relates to the maximum sample size and ignores the fact that the sample size is a random variable, as the study could be stopped early for success. The average sample size ASN introduced in Section 5.2.1 is a more realistic measure and is displayed in the bottom table of the gsd.OF summary output shown above. It displays the boundary crossing probabilities at each interim analysis and the expected sample size E(N) assuming any cross stops the trial under the null and the alternative hypothesis. If there is no treatment effect, the average sample size of 476 is slightly lower than the maximum sample size of 478 patients. However, under the alternative the advantage of group sequential designs becomes evident, as the average sample size is reduced to 358 patients, almost 25% less than in a fixed design. It should be remembered,

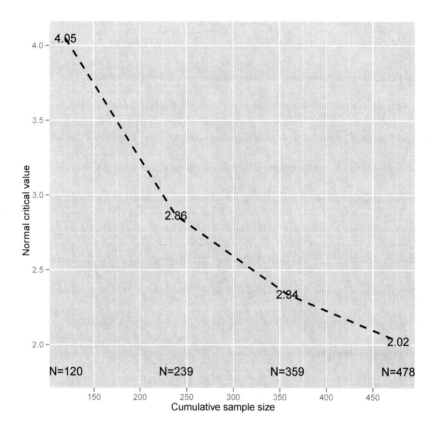

Figure 5.5 Upper stopping boundaries for the O'Brien-Fleming design used in the numerical example.

however, that the computations assume normally distributed outcomes with known variance. These are approximate results that should be viewed with caution if the sample sizes are small.

The previous considerations can be extended by using the `gsProbability` function. This function computes boundary crossing probabilities and expected sample size of a design for arbitrary user-specified treatment effects, bounds, and interim analysis sample sizes. Accordingly, we can call

```
R> gsd.OF3 <- gsProbability(theta = gsd.OF$delta*seq(0,2,0.25),
+                              d = gsd.OF)
R> gsd.OF3
```

One-sided group sequential design with
90 % power and 2.5 % Type I Error.

Analysis   N   Z   Nominal p   Spend

```
        1 120 4.05      0.0000 0.0000
        2 239 2.86      0.0021 0.0021
        3 359 2.34      0.0097 0.0083
        4 478 2.02      0.0215 0.0145
    Total                      0.0250
++ alpha spending:
 O'Brien-Fleming boundary


Boundary crossing probabilities and expected sample size
assume any cross stops the trial

Upper boundary (power or Type I Error)
          Analysis
   Theta       1        2        3        4 Total E{N}
  0.0000 0.0000 0.0021 0.0083 0.0145 0.025   476
  0.0375 0.0001 0.0111 0.0429 0.0700 0.124   470
  0.0750 0.0006 0.0437 0.1395 0.1811 0.365   450
  0.1125 0.0024 0.1281 0.2924 0.2569 0.680   411
  0.1500 0.0080 0.2850 0.4031 0.2040 0.900   358
  0.1875 0.0227 0.4910 0.3752 0.0931 0.982   307
  0.2250 0.0558 0.6745 0.2428 0.0251 0.998   267
  0.2625 0.1188 0.7648 0.1123 0.0041 1.000   239
  0.3000 0.2202 0.7416 0.0378 0.0004 1.000   217
```

for the grid of θ values

```
R> gsd.OF3$theta
```

```
[1] 0.0000 0.0375 0.0750 0.1125 0.1500 0.1875 0.2250 0.2625
[9] 0.3000
```

to obtain a better understanding of the operating characteristics for the selected design.

In addition, the **gsDesign** provides extensive plotting capabilities. Several plot types are available and each of them highlights a different aspect of the selected design. Figure 5.5 shows the default plot by displaying the O'Brien-Fleming stopping boundaries. We now present two further relevant plots. Figure 5.6 displays the cumulative boundary crossing probabilities (i.e., power) separately for the three interim analyses and the final analysis as a function of the treatment effects. Note that the x-axis is scaled relative to the effect size delta for which the trial is powered. Finally, Figure 5.7 displays the average sample sizes by treatment difference (same scale for the x-axis as in Figure 5.6). The horizontal line indicates the sample size of 467 for a comparable fixed design without interim analyses.

The **gsDesign** provides more functionalities than presented here. For example, conditional power can be computed for evaluating interim trends in a group sequential design, but may also be used to adapt a trial design at an interim analysis using the methods of Müller and Schäfer (2001). The gsCP function provides the basis for applying these adaptive methods by computing

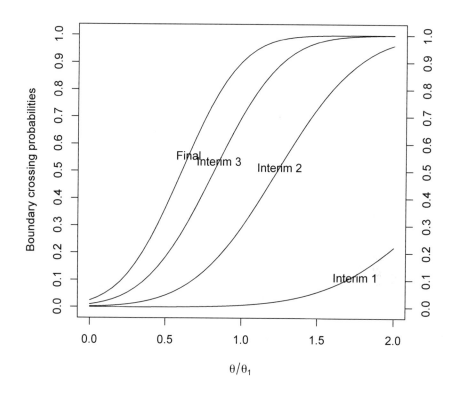

Figure 5.6 Cumulative boundary crossing probabilities for the O'Brien-Fleming design used in the numerical example.

the conditional probability of future boundary crossing given the interim analysis results. The **gsDesign** package can also be used with decision theoretic methods to derive optimal designs. Anderson (2010) describe, for example, the application of Bayesian computations to update the probability of a successful trial based on knowing a bound has not been crossed, but without knowledge of unblinded treatment results. We conclude this section by referring to the **AGSDest** package in R(Hack and Brannath 2009), which allows the computation of repeated confidence intervals as well as confidence intervals based on the stagewise ordering in group sequential designs and adaptive group sequential designs; see Mehta, Bauer, Posch, and Brannath (2007) and Brannath, Mehta, and Posch (2009a) for the technical background.

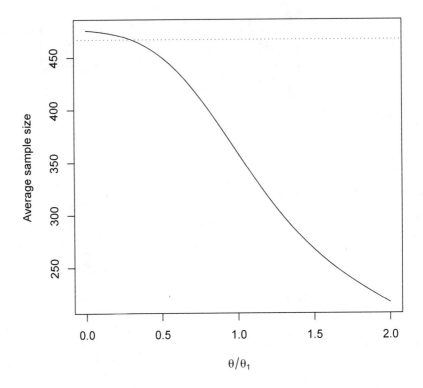

Figure 5.7   Average sample sizes by treatment difference for the O'Brien-Fleming design used in the numerical example. The horizontal line indicates the sample size of a comparable fixed design.

5.2.2 Adaptive designs

Adaptive designs use accumulating data of an ongoing trial to decide on how to modify design aspects without undermining the validity and integrity of the trial. If appropriate methods are used, adaptive designs provide more flexibility than the group sequential designs described in Section 5.2.1 while controlling the Type I error rate. For this reason, adaptive designs providing confirmatory evidence have gained much attention in recent years. Especially in the drug development area the expectation has arisen that carefully planned and conducted studies based on adaptive designs help increasing the efficiency by making better use of the observed data.

There is a rich literature on such approaches for trials with a single null hypothesis, including p-value combination methods (Bauer and Köhne 1994), self-designing trials (Fisher 1998), and methods based on the conditional error function (Proschan and Hunsberger 1995; Müller and Schäfer 2001). In this section, we consider adaptive designs with multiple hypotheses. Bauer and Kieser (1999) proposed an analysis method for adaptive designs involving treatment selection at interim. Kieser, Bauer, and Lehmacher (1999) used a similar approach in the context of multiple outcome variables. Hommel (2001) subsequently formulated a general framework to select and add hypotheses in an adaptive design. Posch, König, Branson, Brannath, Dunger-Baldauf, and Bauer (2005) derived simultaneous confidence intervals and adjusted p-values for adaptive designs with treatment selection. In the sequel, we follow the description of Bretz, Schmidli, König, Racine, and Maurer (2006) and show how to test adaptively multiple hypotheses by applying p-value combination methods to closed test procedures. We refer to Bretz, König, Brannath, Glimm, and Posch (2009a) and the references therein for details on adaptive designs providing confirmatory evidence.

Basic theory

For simplicity, we start considering a single one-sided null hypothesis H in a two-stage design, that is, with one single interim analysis. Based on the data from the first stage it is decided at the interim analysis, whether the study is continued (conducting the second stage) or not (early stopping either due to futility or due to early rejection of H). In case that one continues with the second stage, the final analysis at the end of the study combines the results of both stages. Let p_j denote the p-value for stage $j = 1, 2$. Following Bauer and Köhne (1994), an adaptive design is specified as follows:

(i) Define a test procedure for stage 1, determine the stopping rules for the interim decision and pre-specify a combination function $C = C(p_1, p_2)$ of p_1 and p_2 for the final analysis.

(ii) Conduct stage 1 of the study, resulting in p_1.

(iii) Based on p_1, decide whether to stop at interim (either rejecting or retaining H) or to continue the study.

(iv) If the study is continued, use all information (also external to the study, if available) to design the second stage, such as reassessing the stage 2 sample size.

(v) Conduct stage 2 of the study, resulting in p_2 with p_1 being independent of p_2 under H.

(vi) Combine p_1 and p_2 using C and test H by comparing C with an appropriate critical value.

Adaptive designs offer a high degree of flexibility during the conduct of the trial. Among multistage designs, they require the least amount of decision rule pre-specification prior to a study. Furthermore, the total information available at the interim analysis can be used in designing the second stage.

Different possibilities exist to combine the data from both stages. A common choice is Fisher's combination test which rejects H at the final stage if

$$C(p_1, p_2) = p_1 p_2 \leq c = \exp(-\chi^2_{4,1-\alpha}/2),$$

where $\chi^2_{\nu,1-\alpha}$ denotes the critical value of the χ^2 distribution with ν degrees of freedom at level $1 - \alpha$ (Bauer and Köhne 1994). Assume that early stopping boundaries α_0 and α_1 are available such that (i) if $p_1 \leq \alpha_1$ the trial stops after the interim analysis with an early rejection of H, and (ii) if $p_1 \geq \alpha_0$ the trial stops after the interim analysis for futility (H is retained). In order to maintain the Type I error rate at pre-specified level α simultaneously across both stages, α_1 is computed by solving $\alpha_1 + c(\ln \alpha_0 - \ln \alpha_1) = \alpha$ for given α and α_0. Note that if $\alpha_0 = 1$ no stopping for futility is foreseen and if $\alpha_1 = 0$ no early rejection of H is possible.

Another popular choice is the weighted inverse normal combination function

$$C(p_1, p_2) = 1 - \Phi \left[w_1 \, \Phi^{-1}(1 - p_1) + w_2 \, \Phi^{-1}(1 - p_2) \right],$$

where w_1 and w_2 denote pre-specified weights such that $w_1^2 + w_2^2 = 1$ and Φ denotes the cumulative distribution function of the standard normal distribution (Lehmacher and Wassmer 1999; Cui, Hung, and Wang 1999). Note that for the one-sided test of the mean of normally distributed observations with known variance, the inverse normal combination test with pre-planned stage-wise sample sizes n_1, n_2 and weights $w_1^2 = n_1/(n_1 + n_2)$, $w_2^2 = n_2/(n_1 + n_2)$ is equivalent to a classical two-stage group sequential test if no adaptations are performed (the term in squared brackets is simply the standardized to-tal mean). Thus, the quantities α_1, α_0 and c required for the inverse normal method can be computed with standard software for group sequential trials; see Section 5.2.1.

We now consider the case of testing m elementary null hypotheses $H_1, \ldots, H_m$. To make the ideas concrete, we assume the comparison of m treatments with a control, although the methodology reviewed below holds more generally and covers many other applications; see Schmidli, Bretz, Racine, and Maurer (2006); Wang, O'Neill, and Hung (2007); and Brannath, Zuber, Branson, Bretz, Gallo, Posch, and Racine-Poon (2009b) for examples. Let $H_i : \theta_i \leq 0, i = 1, \ldots, m$, denote the related m one-sided null hypotheses, where θ_i denotes the mean effect difference of treatment i against control. The general rule is to apply the closure principle from Section 2.2.3 by constructing all intersection hypotheses and to test each of them with a suitable combination test (Bauer and Kieser 1999; Kieser et al. 1999; Hommel 2001). Following the closure principle, a null hypothesis H_i is rejected if all intersection hypotheses contained in H_i are also rejected by their combination tests. Consider Figure 5.8 for an example of testing adaptively $m = 2$ hypotheses. Let H_1 and H_2 denote the elementary hypotheses and H_{12} the single intersection hypothesis to be tested according to the closure principle. Let further $p_{i,j}$ denote the one-sided p-value for hypothesis $H_i, i \in \{1, 2, 12\}$, at stage $j = 1, 2$. Finally, let $C(p_{i,1}, p_{i,2}), i \in \{1, 2, 12\}$, denote the combination function C applied to the p-values $p_{i,j}$ from stage $j = 1, 2$. Note that different combination functions as well as different stopping boundaries could be used within the closed hypotheses set (for simplicity we omit this generalization here). According to the closure principle, H_1 (say) is rejected at familywise error rate α, if H_1 and H_{12} are both rejected at level α. That is, H_1 is rejected if $C(p_{1,1}, p_{1,2}) \leq c_1$ and $C(p_{12,1}, p_{12,2}) \leq c_{12}$, where c_1 and c_{12} are suitable critical values, as described above.

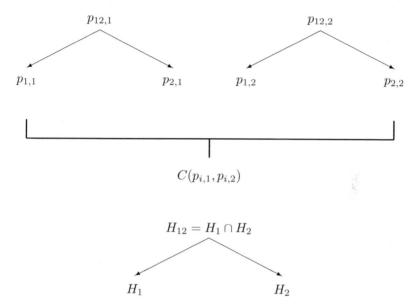

Figure 5.8 Schematic diagram of the closure principle for testing adaptively two null hypotheses H_1 and H_2 and their intersection.

An example

In this section we use a numerical example to illustrate the above methodology with the **asd** package, which supports the design of adaptive trials in R. For details on **asd** we refer to Parsons, Friede, Todd, Valdes-Marquez, Chataway, Nicholas, and Stallard (2010) and the manual accompanying the package (Parsons 2010). For adaptive designs involving a single null hypothesis one can alternatively use the **adaptTest** package in R(Vandemeulebroecke 2009).

The asd.sim function from the **asd** package runs simulations for a trial design that tests a number of treatments against a single control. Test treatments are compared to the control treatment using the Dunnett test from Section 4.1. An interim analysis is undertaken using an early outcome measure, assumed to be normally distributed, and characterized by standardized treatment effects with variances assumed to be equal to one, for each treatment (and control). A decision is made on which of the treatments to take

forward, using a pre-defined selection rule. Data are simulated for the final
outcome measure, also characterized by standardized treatment effects, with
variance assumed equal to one and a fixed correlation between the final and
the early outcomes. Data from the interim and final analyses for the final outcome measure are combined together using either the inverse normal or Fisher
combination test and hypotheses are tested at the selected level.

For illustration, suppose that we plan an adaptive trial design to compare
$m = 2$ dose levels with placebo for a normal distributed outcome variable. Assume that we target at 90% power to detect a standardized treatment effect
size of 0.3 to compare patients under treatment (one of the two dose levels)
and control (placebo). For simplicity, we assume further that at the interim
analysis we already observe the final outcome measure and we select the treatment with the larger observed effect size for the second stage. Assuming equal
treatment effect sizes and a pre-planned group sample size of 110 patients per
stage, we can call

```
R> library("asd")
R> res <- asd.sim(nsamp = c(110, 110), early = c(0.3, 0.3),
+        final = c(0.3, 0.3), nsim = 10000, corr = 1, select = 1,
+        ptest = c(1, 2))
R> res
$count.total
      1 2
n 10000 0

$select.total
      1    2
n 4996 5004

$reject.total
    H1    H2
n 4525 4496

$sim.reject
  Total
n  9021
```

In this call, `early = c(0.3, 0.3)` and `final = c(0.3, 0.3)` specify the
vectors with the standardized treatment effects for the early and the final
outcome variable, respectively. Further, the correlation `corr = 1` between the
early and final outcome measure reflects the fact that at the interim analysis
we already observe the final outcome measure. The `select = 1` option ensures
that we select the treatment with the larger observed effect size for the second
stage. Finally, `ptest = c(1, 2)` will count rejections for testing treatments
1 and 2 against control.

We conclude from the output that each treatment has a chance of 50%
to be selected for the second stage, as seen from `res$select.total`. Further, `res$reject.total` gives the individual power of about 45% to reject

a selected treatment at study end and `res$sim.reject` gives the disjunctive power of about 90% to declare any of the two effective treatments significantly better than placebo (recall Section 2.1.1 for an overview of power in multiple hypotheses testing).

In practice, when designing a real clinical trial, uncertainty about the true effect sizes and other parameters exist. In addition, the interim decision rule of selecting the better of the two doses may not apply because of unforeseen safety signals. Extensive clinical trial simulations have therefore to be conducted to investigate the operating characteristics of an adaptive design (Bretz and Wang 2010).

To give an example of what could be done at the planning stage, we investigate in Figure 5.9 the disjunctive power as a function of θ_1 for different designs options:

(A) select the best treatment (`select = 1`),

(B) select both treatments (`select = 2`), and

(C) select randomly one of the two treatments at the interim analysis (`select = 5`).

Further design options are available with the **asd** package but will not be considered here. Note that the total sample size n is not the same for the three options. For example, we have $n = 3 \times 110 + 3 \times 110 = 660$ for option (B), but only $n = 3 \times 110 + 2 \times 110 = 550$ for option (A). Although the unequal total sample sizes makes it difficult to compare the three options, Figure 5.9 reflects current practice of calculating sample sizes and is therefore of relevance. With the methods implemented in **asd**, sample size reallocation could be applied to ensure a constant total sample size. For illustration, we include in Figure 5.9 design option (D) that selects the best treatment at the interim analysis and performs a sample size reallocation for the second stage such that we have $330/2 = 165$ patients for the two remaining treatment arms (selected treatment and control).

We conclude from Figure 5.9 that design option (C) is considerably less powerful than the competing designs. This is not surprising, as for small values of θ_1 there is a chance that the truly inferior treatment is selected with option (C). As mentioned above, however, unforeseen safety signals may in practice lead to the selection of the treatment with the smaller observed interim effect, which may lead to a potentially substantial reduction in power, as seen in Figure 5.9. Options (A) and (B) have similar power performances, although option (A) saves about 16% of sample size, which will be perceived as an efficiency gain. As expected, option (D) is more powerful than option (A) because of the additional 110 patients in the second stage. Interestingly, comparing options (B) and (D) reveals that for a given constant total sample size selecting the better of the two treatments at the interim analysis leads to considerably higher power than continuing with both treatments in the second stage.

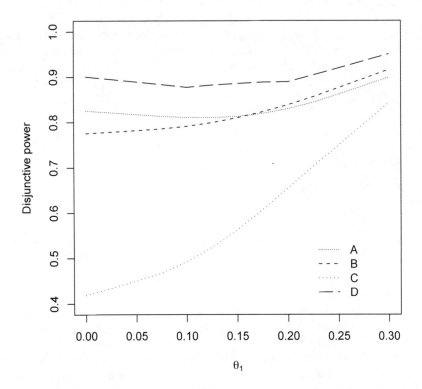

Figure 5.9 Disjunctive power for four design options: (A) select the best treatment without sample size reallocation, (B) select both treatments,
(C) select randomly one of the two treatments, and (D) select the
best treatment with sample size reallocation.

5.3 Combination of multiple comparison procedures with modeling techniques

In Section 4.3 we described a variety of powerful trend tests to detect significant dose response signals. Using these methods, we can assess whether or not
changes in dose lead to desirable changes in an (efficacy or safety) outcome
variable of interest. Once such a dose response signal has been shown (that
is, the so-called *proof-of-concept* (PoC) has been established), the question of
what comprises a "good" dose arises. To address this question, stepwise test
procedures based on the closure principle can be used. To mention only a few
papers, we refer the reader to Tamhane, Hochberg, and Dunnett (1996); Bauer
(1997); Hsu and Berger (1999); Tamhane, Dunnett, Green, and Wetherington

(2001); Bretz et al. (2003), and Strassburger et al. (2007), which all address different aspects of dose finding using multiple comparison procedures; see also Tamhane and Logan (2006) for a review.

Multiple comparison procedures regard the dose as a qualitative factor and generally make few, if any, assumptions about the underlying dose response relationship. However, inferences about the target dose are restricted to the discrete, possibly small set of doses used in the trial. On the other hand, modeling approaches can be used which assume a parametric (typically non-linear) functional relationship between dose and response. The dose is assumed to be a quantitative factor, allowing greater flexibility for estimating a target dose. But its validity depends on an appropriately pre-specified dose response model for the final analysis. In this section we describe a hybrid methodology combining multiple comparison procedures with modeling techniques, denoted as MCP-Mod procedure (Bretz, Pinheiro, and Branson 2005). This approach maintains the flexibility of modeling dose response relationships, while preserving robustness with respect to model misspecification through the use of appropriate multiple comparison procedures.

In Section 5.3.1, we describe the MCP-Mod procedure in more detail. To illustrate the methodology, we analyze in Section 5.3.2 a dose response study and describe the **DoseFinding** package (Bornkamp, Pinheiro, and Bretz 2010), which allows one to design and analyze dose finding studies using the MCP-Mod procedure.

5.3.1 MCP-Mod: Dose response analyses under model uncertainty

The motivation for MCP-Mod is based on the work by Tukey, Ciminera, and Heyse (1985), who recognized that the power of standard dose response trend tests depends on the (unknown) dose response relationship. They proposed to simultaneously use several trend tests and subsequently adjust the resulting p-values for multiplicity. Related ideas were also proposed by Westfall (1997) and Stewart and Ruberg (2000), who all use contrast tests and aim at letting the contrast coefficients mirror potential dose response shapes. Bretz, Pinheiro, and Branson (2004); Bretz et al. (2005) formalized these ideas, leading to the MCP-Mod procedure described below. We refer to Pinheiro, Bornkamp, and Bretz (2006a) for advice on design issues when planning a dose finding experiment using MCP-Mod and Dette, Bretz, Pepelyshev, and Pinheiro (2008) for related optimal designs under model uncertainty. This section can be viewed as a continuation of the discussion started in Section 4.3, where we described the approach from Westfall (1997) and contrasted it with the trend tests from Williams (1971) and Marcus (1976). Note that the theoretical framework from Chapter 3 also applies to the MCP-Mod procedure, thus leading to a powerful method combining multiple comparisons and modeling in general parametric models.

We begin with an overview of the MCP-Mod procedure in Figure 5.10, which has several steps. The procedure starts by defining a set $\mathcal{M}$ of candidate models covering a suitable range of dose response shapes. Each of the dose response shapes in the candidate set is tested using optimal contrasts and employing a max-t test of the form (2.1) while controlling the familywise error rate. A dose response signal (i.e., PoC) is established when at least one of the model tests is significant. Once PoC is verified, either a "best" model or a weighted average over the set of models corrsponding to the significant contrasts is used to estimate the dose response profile and the target doses of interest.

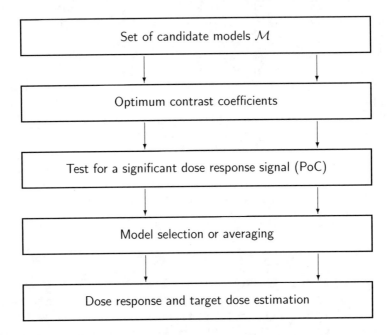

Figure 5.10   Schematic overview of the MCP-Mod procedure.

Below, we assume that we observe a response y for a given set of parallel groups of subjects corresponding to doses $d_2, d_3, \ldots, d_k$ plus placebo d_1, for a total of k arms. For the purpose of testing a dose response signal and estimating target doses, we consider the one-way layout

$$y_{ij} = \mu_{d_i} + \epsilon_{ij}, \tag{5.1}$$

where $\mu_{d_i} = f(d_i)$ denotes the mean response at dose d_i for some dose response model $f(.)$, n_i denotes the number of subjects allocated to dose d_i, $n = \sum_{i=1}^{k} n_i$ denotes the total sample size, and $\varepsilon_{ij} \sim N(0, \sigma^2)$ denotes the error term for subject $j = 1, \ldots, n_i$, within dose group $i = 1, \ldots, k$. Following Bretz et al. (2005), we note that most parametric dose response models $f(d, \boldsymbol{\theta})$ used in practice can be written as

$$f(d, \boldsymbol{\theta}) = \theta_0 + \theta_1 f^0(d, \boldsymbol{\theta}^*), \tag{5.2}$$

where $f^0(d, \boldsymbol{\theta}^*)$ denotes the standardized model, parameterized by the vector $\boldsymbol{\theta}^*$. In this parametrization, θ_0 is a location and θ_1 is a scale parameter, so only the parameter $\boldsymbol{\theta}^*$ determines the shape of the model function. For the derivation of optimal contrasts further below it is sufficient to use the standardized model f^0 instead of the full model f, which motivates the reparametrization in (5.2).

Table 5.6 summarizes a selection of linear and non-linear regression models frequently used to represent dose response relationships, together with their respective standardized versions. A common problem is the specification of the model contrasts based on knowledge about the standardized model parameters $\boldsymbol{\theta}^*$ before study begins. Such best guesses ("guesstimates") are typically derived from available information of the expected percentage p^* of the maximum response associated with a given dose d^*. We refer to Pinheiro, Bretz, and Branson (2006b) for strategies to elicit the necessary information.

Assume that a set $\mathcal{M}$ of M parameterized candidate models is given, with corresponding model functions $f_m(d, \boldsymbol{\theta}_m), m = 1, \ldots, M$, and parameters $\boldsymbol{\theta}_m^*$ of the standardized models f^0, which determine the model shapes. Each of the dose response models in the candidate set is tested using a single contrast test statistic

$$t_m = \frac{\sum_{i=1}^{k} c_{mi}\bar{x}_i}{s\sqrt{\sum_{i=1}^{k} c_{mi}^2/n_i}}, \quad m = 1, \ldots, M,$$

where $s^2 = \sum_{i=1}^{k} \sum_{j=1}^{n_i} (x_{ij} - \bar{x}_i)^2/(n - k)$ is the pooled variance estimate and $c_{m1}, \ldots, c_{mk}$ denote contrast coefficients subject to $\sum_{i=1}^{k} c_{mi} = 0$. As described below, the contrast coefficients $c_{m1}, \ldots, c_{mk}$ are chosen to maximize the power of detecting the m-th model. Every single contrast test thus translates into a decision procedure to determine whether the given dose response shape is statistically significant, based on the observed data.

It can be shown that the optimal contrast coefficients for detecting the m-th model depend only on the model shape, that is, only on the parameters of the standardized models f^0. Letting

$$(\mu_{m1}^0, \ldots, \mu_{mk}^0) = (f_m^0(d_1, \boldsymbol{\theta}_m^*), \ldots, f_m^0(d_k, \boldsymbol{\theta}_m^*)),$$

the i-th entry of the optimal contrast $\mathbf{c}_m$ for detecting the shape m is proportional to

$$n_i(\mu_{mi}^0 - \bar{\mu}), \quad i = 1, \ldots, k,$$

where $\bar{\mu} = n^{-1} \sum_{i=1}^{k} \mu_{mi}^0 n_i$ (Bretz et al. 2005; Bornkamp 2006). A unique representation of the optimal contrast can be obtained by imposing the constraint $\sum_{i=1}^{k} c_{mi}^2 = 1$.

The detection of a significant dose response signal is based on the max-t test statistic

$$t_{\max} = \max\{t_1, \ldots, t_M\}.$$

Under the null hypothesis of no dose response effect, $\mu_{d_1} = \ldots = \mu_{d_k}$, and the distributional assumptions stated in (5.1) it follows that $t_1, \ldots, t_M$ are jointly

Name	$f(d, \boldsymbol{\theta})$	$f^0(d, \boldsymbol{\theta}^*)$
linear	$E_0 + \delta d$	d
linlog	$E_0 + \delta \log(d + c)$	$\log(d + c)$
quadratic	$E_0 + \beta_1 d + \beta_2 d^2$	$d + \delta d^2$ if $\beta_2 < 0$
emax	$E_0 + E_{\max} d/(ED_{50} + d)$	$d/(ED_{50} + d)$
logistic	$E_0 + E_{\max}/\{1 + \exp[(ED_{50} - d)/\delta]\}$	$1/\{1 + \exp[(ED_{50} - d)/\delta]\}$
exponential	$E_0 + E_1(\exp(d/\delta) - 1)$	$\exp(d/\delta) - 1$
sigEmax	$E_0 + E_{\max} d^h/(ED_{50}^h + d^h)$	$d^h/(ED_{50}^h + d^h)$
betaMod	$E_0 + E_{\max} B(\delta_1, \delta_2)(d/D)^{\delta_1}(1 - d/D)^{\delta_2}$	$B(\delta_1, \delta_2)(d/D)^{\delta_1}(1 - d/D)^{\delta_2}$

Table 5.6   Dose response models implemented in the **DoseFinding** package. For the beta model $B(\delta_1, \delta_2) = (\delta_1 + \delta_2)^{\delta_1 + \delta_2}/(\delta_1^{\delta_1}\delta_2^{\delta_2})$ and for the quadratic model $\delta = \frac{\beta_2}{|\beta_1|}$. For the quadratic model the standardized model function is given for the concave-shaped form.

multivariate t distributed with $n-k$ degrees of freedom and correlation matrix $\mathbf{R} = (\rho_{ij})_{ij}$, where

$$\rho_{ij} = \frac{\sum_{l=1}^{k} c_{il} c_{jl}/n_l}{\sqrt{\sum_{l=1}^{k} c_{il}^2/n_l \sum_{l=1}^{k} c_{jl}^2/n_l}}.$$

Note that the description above parallels the development of multiple comparison procedures for the general linear models in Section 3.1, and, more broadly speaking, for the general parametric models in Section 3.2. Numerical integration methods to calculate the required multivariate t (or, if required, normal) probabilities are implemented in the **mvtnorm** package (Hothorn et al. 2001); see Genz and Bretz (1999, 2002, 2009) for the mathematical details.

Proof-of-concept is established if $t_{\max} \geq u_{1-\alpha}$, where $u_{1-\alpha}$ denotes the multiplicity adjusted critical value at level $1 - \alpha$ from the multivariate t distribution. Furthermore, all dose response shapes with associated contrast test statistics larger than $u_{1-\alpha}$ can be declared statistically significant at level $1 - \alpha$ under a strong control of the familywise error rate. These models then form a reference set $\mathcal{M}^* = \{M_1, \ldots, M_L\} \subseteq \mathcal{M}$ of L significant models. If no contrast test is statistically significant, the procedure stops indicating that a dose response relationship cannot be established from the observed data.

If a significant dose response signal is established, the next step is to estimate the dose response curve and the target doses of interest. This can be achieved by either selecting a single model out of $\mathcal{M}^*$ or applying model averaging techniques to $\mathcal{M}^*$. A common target dose of interest is the minimum effective dose (MED), which is defined as the smallest dose ensuring a clinically relevant and statistically significant improvement over placebo (Ruberg 1995a). Formally,

$$\text{MED} = \min\{d \in (d_1, d_k] : f(d) > f(d_1) + \Delta\},$$

where Δ is a given relevance threshold. A common estimate for the MED is

$$\widehat{\text{MED}} = \min\{d \in (d_1, d_k] : \hat{f}(d) > \hat{f}(0) + \Delta, L(d) > \hat{f}(0)\}$$

where $\hat{f}(d)$ is the predicted response at dose d, and $U(d)$ and $L(d)$ are the corresponding pointwise confidence intervals of level $1 - 2\gamma$. The choice of γ is not driven by the purpose of controlling Type I error rates, in contrast to the selection of α for controlling the familywise error rate in the PoC declaration. Other estimates are possible and we refer to Bretz et al. (2005) for further details.

Several possibilities exist to select a single model from $\mathcal{M}^*$ for the target dose estimation step. Because max-t tests have been used above to detect a significant dose response signal, a natural approach is to select the "most significant" model shape, that is, the one associated with the largest contrast test statistic. Alternatively, standard information criteria like the AIC or BIC might be used. The estimate of the model function is obtained by maximizing the likelihood of the model with respect to its parameters $\boldsymbol{\theta}$.

An alternative to selecting a single dose response model is to apply model averaging and produce weighted estimates across all models in $\mathcal{M}^*$ for a given quantity ψ of interest. In dose response analyses, the parameter ψ could be either a target dose of interest (such as the MED) or the mean responses at specific doses $d \in [d_1, d_k]$. Buckland, Burnham, and Augustin (1997) proposed using the weighted estimate

$$\widehat{\psi} = \sum_\ell w_\ell \widehat{\psi_\ell},$$

where ψ has the same meaning under all models and $\widehat{\psi_\ell}$ is the estimate of ψ under model ℓ for given probabilities w_ℓ. The idea is to use estimates for the final data analysis which rely on the averaged estimates across all L models. Buckland et al. (1997) proposed using of the weights

$$w_\ell = \frac{\exp(-\frac{\text{IC}_\ell}{2})}{\sum_{j=1}^L \exp(-\frac{\text{IC}_j}{2})}, \quad \ell = 1, \ldots, L,$$

which are dependent on a common information criterion IC, such as AIC or BIC applied to each of the L models.

5.3.2 A dose response example

To illustrate the MCP-Mod procedure we use the `biom` dose response data from Bretz et al. (2005). The data are from a randomized double-blind parallel group trial with a total of 100 patients allocated to either placebo or one of four active doses coded as 0.05, 0.20, 0.60, and 1, with 20 patients per group. The clinical threshold is $\Delta = 0.4$, the significance level is $\alpha = 0.05$ and the dose estimation model is selected according to the maximum test statistic. We use the **DoseFinding** package to perform the computations. A detailed description of this package is given in Bornkamp, Pinheiro, and Bretz (2009).

As described in Section 5.3.1, the MCP-Mod procedure starts by defining a set $\mathcal{M}$ of candidate models covering a suitable range of dose response shapes. The candidate set of models needs to be constructed as a list, where the list elements should be named as the underlying dose response model function (see Table 5.6) and the individual list entries should correspond to the specified guesstimates. Suppose we want to include in our candidate set a linear model, an $\text{E}_{\max}$ model and a logistic model. Concluding from the standardized model functions in Table 5.6 we need to specify one value for the $\text{E}_{\max}$ model shape (for the ED_{50} parameter), two values for the logistic model shape (for the ED_{50} and δ parameters) but no guesstimate for the linear model as its standardized model function does not contain an unknown parameter. These guesstimates are used below for the calculation of optimal contrast coefficients. Suppose our guesstimate for the ED_{50} parameter of the $\text{E}_{\max}$ model is 0.2, while the guesstimate for (ED_{50}, δ) for the logistic model is $(0.4, 0.09)$. The model list is then defined through

```
R> library("DoseFinding")
R> candMods <- list(linear = NULL, emax = 0.2,
+        logistic = c(0.25, 0.09))
```

We visualize the model shapes from the candidate set with the `plotModels` function. As the candidate model shapes do not determine the location (baseline effect) and scale (maximum effect) of the model, we also need to specify those parameters via the `base` and `maxEff` arguments. Using the candidate set `candMods` from above, we define a vector for the dose levels and then call `plotModels`,

```
R> doses <- c(0, 0.05, 0.2, 0.6, 1)
R> plotModels(candMods, doses, base = 0, maxEff = 1)
```

see Figure 5.11 for the plot.

After these preparations, we can now use the `MCPMod` function, which implements the full MCP-Mod procedure. Thus, we can call

```
R> data("biom", package = "DoseFinding")
R> res <- MCPMod(resp ~ dose, biom, candMods, alpha = 0.05,
+        pVal = TRUE, clinRel = 0.4)
```

to run the MCP-Mod procedure. In the previous call the arguments to the `MCPMod` function are mostly self-explanatory; the `pVal = TRUE` options specifies that multiplicity adjusted p-values for the max-t test should be calculated.

A brief summary of the results is available via the `print` method for the `MCPMod` objects

```
R> res
```

MCPMod

PoC (alpha = 0.05, one-sided): yes
Model with highest t-statistic: emax
Model used for dose estimation: emax
Dose estimate:
MED2,80%
    0.17

We conclude from the `PoC` line that there is significant dose response signal, which means that the max-t test is significant at the one-sided significance level $\alpha = 0.05$. Additionally, the E_{max} contrast has the largest test statistic and consequently the E_{max} model was used for the dose estimation step. The MED estimate is 0.17.

A more detailed summary of the results is available via the `summary` method

```
R> summary(res)
```

MCPMod

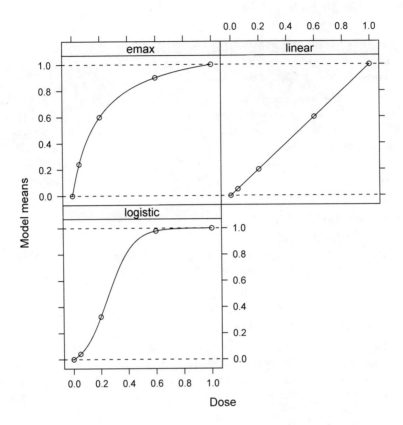

Figure 5.11   Model shapes for the selected candidate model set.

```
Input parameters:
 alpha = 0.05
 alternative: one.sided, one sided
 model selection: maxT
 clinical relevance = 0.4
 dose estimator: MED2 (gamma = 0.1)
 optimizer: nls

Optimal Contrasts:
      linear    emax logistic
0    -0.437 -0.643   -0.478
0.05 -0.378 -0.361   -0.435
0.2  -0.201  0.061   -0.147
0.6   0.271  0.413    0.519
1     0.743  0.530    0.540
```

```
Contrast Correlation:
         linear  emax logistic
linear    1.000 0.912    0.945
emax      0.912 1.000    0.956
logistic  0.945 0.956    1.000

Multiple Contrast Test:
         Tvalue pValue
emax       3.46  0.001
logistic   3.23  0.002
linear     2.97  0.003

Selected for dose estimation:
  emax

Parameter estimates:
emax model:
  e0   eMax   ed50
0.322 0.746 0.142

Dose estimate
MED2,80%
   0.17
```

From the output above, we first obtain some information about important input parameters that were used when performing the MCP-Mod procedure. Then the output displays the optimal contrasts and their correlations. The contrast test statistics, their multiplicity adjusted p-values and the critical value are shown in the next table. Finally, the output contains information about the fitted dose response model, its parameter estimates and the target dose estimate. The core results are of course the same as the results displayed earlier with the print method.

A graphical display of the dose response model used for dose estimation can be obtained via the plot method for MCPMod objects,

```
R> plot(res, complData = TRUE, clinRel = TRUE, CI = TRUE,
+        doseEst = TRUE)
```

The resulting plot is shown in Figure 5.12. The options complData, CI, clinRel, and doseEst specify, which of the following should be included in the plot when set to TRUE: the full dose response dataset (instead of displaying only the group means), the confidence intervals for the mean of the function, the clinical relevance threshold and the dose estimate, respectively.

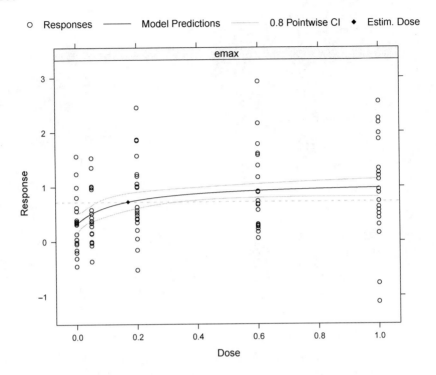

Figure 5.12   Fitted model for the biom data.

Bibliography

Agresti, A., Bini, M., Bertaccini, B., and Ryu, E. (2008), "Simultaneous confidence intervals for comparing binomial parameters," *Biometrics*, 64, 1270–1275. Cited on p. 52.

Altman, D. G. (1991), *Practical Statistics for Medical Research*, London: Chapman & Hall. Cited on p. 3.

Anderson, K. (2010), **gsDesign**: Group Sequential Design, URL `http://CRAN.R-project.org/package=gsDesign`, R package version 2.3. Cited on p. 140, 141, 145, 149.

Armitage, P., McPherson, C. K., and Rowe, B. C. (1969), "Repeated significance tests on accumulating data," *Journal of the Royal Statistical Society, Series A*, 132, 235–244. Cited on p. 142.

Bartholomew, D. J. (1961), "Ordered tests in the analysis of variance," *Biometrika*, 48, 325–332. Cited on p. 103.

Bates, D. and Sarkar, D. (2010), **lme4**: Linear Mixed-Effects Models Using S4 Classes, URL `http://CRAN.R-project.org/package=lme4`, R package version 0.999375-33. Cited on p. 126.

Bauer, P. (1997), "A note on multiple testing procedures in dose finding," *Biometrics*, 53, 1125–1128. Cited on p. 156.

Bauer, P., Hackl, P., Hommel, G., and Sonnemann, E. (1986), "Multiple testing of pairs of one-sided hypotheses," *Metrika*, 33, 121–127. Cited on p. 17.

Bauer, P. and Kieser, M. (1999), "Combining different phases in the development of medical treatments within a single trial," *Statistics in Medicine*, 18, 1833–1848. Cited on p. 151, 152.

Bauer, P. and Köhne, K. (1994), "Evaluation of experiments with adaptive interim analyses," *Biometrics*, 50, 1029–1041. Cited on p. 150, 151, 152.

Bauer, P., Röhmel, J., Maurer, W., and Hothorn, L. (1998), "Testing strategies in multi-dose experiments including active control," *Statistics in Medicine*, 17, 2133–2146. Cited on p. 28.

Benjamini, Y. (2010), "Simultaneous and selective inference: current successes and future challenges," *Biometrical Journal*, (in press). Cited on p. 14.

Benjamini, Y. and Hochberg, Y. (1995), "Controlling the false discovery rate: A practical and powerful approach to multiple testing," *Journal of the Royal Statistical Society, Series B*, 57, 289–300. Cited on p. 13, 61.

Benjamini, Y. and Hochberg, Y. (2000), "On the adaptive control of the false discovery rate in multiple testing with independent statistics," *Journal of Educational and Behavioural Statistics*, 25, 60–83. Cited on p. 35.

Benjamini, Y. and Yekutieli, D. L. (2001), "The control of the false discovery rate in multiple testing under dependency," *The Annals of Statistics*, 29, 1165–1188. Cited on p. 61.

Berger, R. L. (1982), "Multi-parameter hypothesis testing and acceptance sampling," *Technometrics*, 24, 295–300. Cited on p. 22.

Bergmann, B. and Hommel, G. (1988), "Improvements of general multiple test procedures for redundant systems of hypotheses," in *Multiple Hypothesenprüfung - Multiple Hypotheses Testing*, eds. P. Bauer, G. Hommel, and E. Sonnemann, Heidelberg: Springer, pp. 100–115. Cited on p. 34, 95.

Bernhard, G. (1992), Computergestützte Durchführung von multiplen Testprozeduren, Universität Mainz, Germany, PhD thesis. Cited on p. 95.

Berry, D. (2007), "The difficult and ubiquitous problems of multiplicities," *Pharmaceutical Statistics*, 6, 155–160. Cited on p. xiv.

Bofinger, E. (1987), "Step down procedures for comparison with a control," *Australian Journal of Statistics*, 29, 348–364. Cited on p. 81.

Bönsch, D., Lederer, T., Reulbach, U., Hothorn, T., Kornhuber, J., and Bleich, S. (2005), "Joint analysis of the NACP-REP1 marker within the alpha synuclein gene concludes association with alcohol dependence," *Human Molecular Genetics*, 14, 967–971. Cited on p. 114.

Bornkamp, B. (2006), Comparison of model-based and model-free approaches for the analysis of dose-response studies, Fachbereich Statistik, Universität Dortmund, Germany, Diploma thesis. Cited on p. 159.

Bornkamp, B., Pinheiro, J., and Bretz, F. (2009), "MCPMod - an R package for the design and analysis of dose-finding studies," *Journal of Statistical Software*, 29, 1–23. Cited on p. 162.

Bornkamp, B., Pinheiro, J., and Bretz, F. (2010), **DoseFinding**: Planning and Analyzing Dose Finding Experiments, URL http://CRAN.R-project.org/package=DoseFinding, R package version 0.2-1. Cited on p. 157.

Brannath, W. and Bretz, F. (2010), "Shortcuts for locally consonant closed test procedures," *Journal of the American Statistical Association*, (in press). Cited on p. 20, 28, 135.

Brannath, W., Mehta, C. R., and Posch, M. (2009a), "Exact confidence bounds following adaptive group sequential tests," *Biometrics*, 65, 539–546. Cited on p. 149.

Brannath, W., Zuber, E., Branson, M., Bretz, F., Gallo, P., Posch, M., and Racine-Poon, A. (2009b), "Confirmatory adaptive designs with Bayesian decision tools for a targeted therapy in oncology," *Statistics in Medicine*, 28, 1445–1463. Cited on p. 152.

Bretz, F. (2006), "An extension of the Williams trend test to general unbalanced linear models," *Computational Statistics & Data Analysis*, 50, 1735–1748. Cited on p. 100, 104, 106.

Bretz, F., Hayter, A., and Genz, A. (2001), "Critical point and power calculations for the studentized range test for generally correlated means," *Journal of Statistical Computation and Simulation*, 71, 85–99. Cited on p. 84.

Bretz, F. and Hothorn, L. A. (2003), "Comparison of exact amd resampling based multiple test procedures," *Communications in Statistics - Computation and Simulation*, 32, 461–473. Cited on p. 140.

Bretz, F., Hothorn, L. A., and Hsu, J. C. (2003), "Identifying effective and/or safe doses by stepwise confidence intervals for ratios," *Statistics in Medicine*, 22, 847–858. Cited on p. 30, 157.

Bretz, F., Hothorn, T., and Westfall, P. (2008a), "Multiple comparison procedures in linear models," in *COMPSTAT 2008 - Proceedings in Computational Statistics*, ed. P. Brito, Heidelberg: Physica Verlag, pp. 423–431. Cited on p. 41.

Bretz, F., Hsu, J. C., Pinheiro, J. C., and Liu, Y. (2008b), "Dose finding - a challenge in statistics," *Biometrical Journal*, 50, 480–504. Cited on p. 100.

Bretz, F., König, F., Brannath, W., Glimm, E., and Posch, M. (2009a), "Adaptive designs for confirmatory clinical trials," *Statistics in Medicine*, 28, 1181–1217. Cited on p. 151.

Bretz, F., Maurer, W., Brannath, W., and Posch, M. (2009b), "A graphical approach to sequentially rejective multiple test procedures," *Statistics in Medicine*, 28, 586–604. Cited on p. 28, 35.

Bretz, F., Maurer, W., and Gallo, P. (2009c), "Discussion of some controversial multiple testing problems in regulatory applications by H.M.J. Hung and S.J. Wang," *Journal of Biopharmaceutical Statistics*, 19, 25–34. Cited on p. 7.

Bretz, F., Maurer, W., and Hommel, G. (2010), "Test and power considerations for multiple endpoint analyses using sequentially rejective graphical procedures," *Statistics in Medicine*, (in press). Cited on p. 16, 28.

Bretz, F., Pinheiro, J. C., and Branson, M. (2004), "On a hybrid method in dose finding studies," *Methods of Information in Medicine*, 43, 457–461. Cited on p. 157.

Bretz, F., Pinheiro, J. C., and Branson, M. (2005), "Combining multiple comparisons and modeling techniques in dose-response studies," *Biometrics*, 61, 738–748. Cited on p. 157, 158, 159, 161, 162.

Bretz, F., Schmidli, H., König, F., Racine, A., and Maurer, W. (2006), "Confirmatory seamless phase II/III clinical trials with hypotheses selection at interim: General concepts (with discussion)," *Biometrical Journal*, 48, 623–634. Cited on p. 151.

Bretz, F. and Wang, S. J. (2010), "Recent developments in adaptive designs. Part II: Success probabilities and effect estimates for Phase III development programs via modern protocol design," *Drug Information Journal*, 44, 333–342. Cited on p. 155.

Brown, L. D. (1984), "A note on the Tukey-Kramer procedure for pairwise comparisons of correlated means," in *Design of Experiments: Ranking and Selection (Essays in Honour of Robert E. Bechhofer)*, eds. T. J. Santner and A. C. Tamhane, New York: Marcel Dekker, pp. 1–6. Cited on p. 84.

Buckland, S. T., Burnham, K. P., and Augustin, N. H. (1997), "Model selection: An integral part of inference," *Biometrics*, 53, 603–618. Cited on p. 162.

Bullinger, L., Döhner, K., Bair, E., Fröhlich, S., Schlenk, R. F., Tibshirani, R., Döhner, H., and Pollack, J. R. (2004), "Use of gene-expression profiling to identify prognostic subclasses in adult acute myloid leukemia," *New England Journal of Medicine*, 350, 1605–1616. Cited on p. 124.

Burman, C. F., Sonesson, C., and Guilbaud, O. (2009), "A recycling framework for the construction of Bonferroni-based multiple tests," *Statistics in Medicine*, 28, 739–761. Cited on p. 28.

Calian, V., Li, D., and Hsu, J. C. (2008), "Partitioning to uncover conditions for permutation tests to control multiple testing error rates," *Biometrical Journal*, 50, 756–766. Cited on p. 134.

Chevret, S. (2006), *Statistical Methods for Dose Finding Experiments*, New York: Wiley. Cited on p. 100.

Chuang-Stein, C., Anderson, K., Gallo, P., and Collins, S. (2006), "Sample size re-estimation: A review and recommendations," *Drug Information Journal*, 40, 475–484. Cited on p. 140.

Cui, L., Hung, H. M. J., and Wang, S. (1999), "Modification of sample size in group sequential clinical trials," *Biometrics*, 55, 321–324. Cited on p. 152.

Dalgaard, P. (2002), *Introductory Statistics with R*, New York: Springer. Cited on p. xv, 3.

Dalgaard, P. (2010), **ISwR**: Introductory Statistics with R, URL http://CRAN.R-project.org/package=ISwR, R package version 2.0-5. Cited on p. 3.

Dette, H., Bretz, F., Pepelyshev, A., and Pinheiro, J. C. (2008), "Optimal designs for dose finding studies," *Journal of the American Statistical Association*, 103, 1225–1237. Cited on p. 157.

Dmitrienko, A., Offen, W. W., and Westfall, P. H. (2003), "Gatekeeping strategies for clinical trials that do not require all primary effects to be significant," *Statistics in Medicine*, 22, 2387–2400. Cited on p. 28, 35.

Dmitrienko, A., Tamhane, A. C., and Bretz, F. (2009), *Multiple Testing Problems in Pharmaceutical Statistics*, Boca Raton: Taylor and Francis. Cited on p. xiii.

Dudoit, S. and van der Laan, M. J. (2008), *Multiple Testing Procedures with Applications to Genomics*, New York: Springer. Cited on p. xiii, 12, 127, 137.

Dunnett, C. W. (1955), "A multiple comparison procedure for comparing several treatments with a control," *Journal of the American Statistical Association*, 50, 1096–1121. Cited on p. 72.

Dunnett, C. W. and Tamhane, A. C. (1991), "Step-down multiple tests for comparing treatments with a control in unbalanced one-way layouts," *Statistics in Medicine*, 10, 939–947. Cited on p. 78.

EMEA (2002), CPMP points to consider on multiplicity issues in clinical trials, European Agency for the Evaluation of Medicinal Products, London, URL http://www.emea.europa.eu/pdfs/human/ewp/090899en.pdf. Cited on p. 9.

EMEA (2009), CHMP guideline on clinical development of fixed combination medicinal products, European Agency for the Evaluation of Medicinal Products, London, URL http://www.emea.europa.eu/pdfs/human/ewp/024095enfin.pdf. Cited on p. 22.

Everitt, B. S. and Hothorn, T. (2009), *A Handbook of Statistical Analyses Using R*, Boca Raton, Florida: Chapman & Hall/CRC Press, 2nd edition. Cited on p. xv.

Finner, H. (1988), "Abgeschlossene multiple Spannweitentests," in *Multiple Hypothesenprüfung - Multiple Hypotheses Testing*, eds. P. Bauer, G. Hommel, and E. Sonnemann, Berlin: Springer, pp. 10–32. Cited on p. 93.

Finner, H. (1999), "Stepwise multiple test procedures and control of directional errors," *The Annals of Statistics*, 27, 274–289. Cited on p. 17.

Finner, H., Giani, G., and Strassburger, K. (2006), "Partitioning principle and selection of good populations," *Journal of Statistical Planning and Inference*, 136, 2053–2069. Cited on p. 30.

Finner, H. and Gontscharuk, V. (2009), "Controlling the familywise error rate with plug-in estimator for the proportion of true null hypotheses," *Journal of the Royal Statistical Society, Series B*, 71, 1031–1048. Cited on p. 35.

Finner, H. and Strassburger, K. (2002), "The partitioning principle: A powerful tool in multiple decision theory," *The Annals of Statistics*, 30, 1194–1213. Cited on p. 11, 18, 29, 30.

Finner, H. and Strassburger, K. (2006), "On δ-equivalence with the best in k-sample models," *Journal of the American Statistical Association*, 101, 737–746. Cited on p. 31.

Fisher, L. D. (1998), "Self-designing clinical trials," *Statistics in Medicine*, 17, 1551–1562. Cited on p. 151.

Gabriel, K. R. (1969), "Simultaneous test procedures - some theory of multiple comparisons," *The Annals of Mathematical Statistics*, 40, 224–250. Cited on p. 11, 20, 21.

Garcia, A. L., Wagner, K., Hothorn, T., Koebnick, C., Zunft, H. J. F., and Trippo, U. (2005), "Improved prediction of body fat by measuring skinfold thickness, circumferences, and bone breadths," *Obesity Research*, 13, 626–634. Cited on p. 108.

Genz, A. and Bretz, F. (1999), "Numerical computation of multivariate *t*-probabilities with application to power calculation of multiple contrasts," *Journal of Statistical Computation and Simulation*, 63, 361–378. Cited on p. 44, 51, 161.

Genz, A. and Bretz, F. (2002), "Methods for the computation of multivariate *t*-probabilities," *Journal of Computational and Graphical Statistics*, 11, 950–971. Cited on p. 44, 51, 161.

Genz, A. and Bretz, F. (2009), *Computation of Multivariate Normal and t Probabilities*, volume 195 of *Lecture Note Series*, Heidelberg: Springer. Cited on p. 44, 45, 51, 73, 84, 161.

Genz, A., Bretz, F., and Hothorn, T. (2010), **mvtnorm**: Multivariate Normal and *t* Distribution, URL http://CRAN.R-project.org/package= robustbase, R package version 0.9-91. Cited on p. 63.

Grechanovsky, E. and Hochberg, Y. (1999), "Closed procedures are better and often admit a shortcut," *Journal of Statistical Planning and Inference*, 76, 79–91. Cited on p. 28.

Guilbaud, O. (2008), "Simultaneous confidence regions corresponding to Holm's step-down procedure and other closed-testing procedures," *Biometrical Journal*, 50, 678–692. Cited on p. 19, 34, 81.

Guilbaud, O. (2009), "Alternative confidence regions for Bonferroni-based closed-testing procedures that are not alpha-exhaustive," *Biometrical Journal*, 51, 721–735. Cited on p. 19.

Hack, N. and Brannath, W. (2009), **AGSDest**: Estimation in Adaptive Group Sequential Trials, URL http://CRAN.R-project.org/package=AGSDest, R package version 1.0. Cited on p. 149.

Hayter, A. J. (1984), "A proof of the conjecture that the Tukey-Kramer multiple comparisons procedure is conservative," *The Annals of Statistics*, 12, 61–75. Cited on p. 84.

Hayter, A. J. (1989), "Pairwise comparisons of generally correlated means," *Journal of the American Statistical Association*, 84, 208–213. Cited on p. 84.

Hayter, A. J. (1990), "A one-sided studentized range test for testing against ordered alternatives," *Journal of the American Statistical Association*, 85, 778–785. Cited on p. 85.

Hayter, A. J. and Hsu, J. C. (1994), "On the relationship between stepwise decision procedures and confidence sets," *Journal of the American Statistical Association*, 89, 128–136. Cited on p. 18, 29.

Heiberger, R. M. (2009), **HH**: Statistical Analysis and Data Display: Heiberger and Holland, URL http://CRAN.R-project.org/package=HH, R package version 2.1-32. Cited on p. 65, 90.

Heiberger, R. M. and Holland, B. (2004), *Statistical Analysis and Data Display: An Intermediate Course with Examples in S-Plus, R, and SAS*, New York: Springer. Cited on p. 89, 93.

Heiberger, R. M. and Holland, B. (2006), "Mean-mean multiple comparison displays for families of linear contrasts," *Journal of Computational and Graphical Statistics*, 15, 937–955. Cited on p. 89, 91, 93.

Herberich, E. (2009), Niveau und Güte simultaner parametrischer Inferenzverfahren, Institut für Statistik, Universität München, Germany, Diploma thesis (in German). Cited on p. 52.

Hochberg, E. and Tamhane, A. C. (1987), *Multiple Comparison Procedures*, New York: John Wiley & Sons. Cited on p. xiii, 11, 22, 41, 93.

Hochberg, Y. (1988), "A sharper Bonferroni procedure for multiple significance testing," *Biometrika*, 75, 800–802. Cited on p. 38.

Holm, S. (1979a), "A simple sequentially rejective multiple test procedure," *Scandinavian Journal of Statistics*, 6, 65–70. Cited on p. 17, 19, 28, 31, 32, 33, 35.

Holm, S. (1979b), A stagewise directional test based on t-statistics, Institute of Mathematics, Chalmers University of Technology, Gothenberg, Statistical Research Report 1979-3. Cited on p. 17.

Hommel, G. (1983), "Tests of the overall hypothesis for arbitrary dependence structures," *Biometrical Journal*, 25, 423–430. Cited on p. 37.

Hommel, G. (1988), "A stagewise rejective multiple test procedure based on a modified Bonferroni test," *Biometrika*, 75, 383–386. Cited on p. 36, 38.

Hommel, G. (1989), "A comparison of two modified Bonferroni procedures," *Biometrika*, 76, 624–625. Cited on p. 38.

Hommel, G. (2001), "Adaptive modifications of hypotheses after an interim analysis," *Biometrical Journal*, 43, 581–589. Cited on p. 151, 152.

Hommel, G. and Bernhard, G. (1992), "Multiple hypotheses testing," in *Computational Aspects of Model Choice*, ed. J. Antoch, Heidelberg: Physica, pp. 211–235. Cited on p. 95.

Hommel, G. and Bernhard, G. (1999), "Bonferroni procedures for logically related hypotheses," *Journal of Statistical Planning and Inference*, 82, 119–128. Cited on p. 34, 95.

Hommel, G. and Bretz, F. (2008), "Aesthetics and power considerations in multiple testing – a contradiction?" *Biometrical Journal*, 50, 657–666. Cited on p. 20, 34, 95.

Hommel, G., Bretz, F., and Maurer, W. (2007), "Powerful short-cuts for multiple testing procedures with special reference to gatekeeping strategies," *Statistics in Medicine*, 26, 4063–4073. Cited on p. 28, 35.

Hommel, G. and Hoffmann, T. (1988), "Controlled uncertainty," in *Multiple Hypothesenprüfung - Multiple Hypotheses Testing*, eds. P. Bauer, G. Hommel, and E. Sonnemann, Heidelberg: Springer, pp. 154–161. Cited on p. 13.

Hothorn, T., Bretz, F., and Genz, A. (2001), "On multivariate t and Gauß probabilities in R," *R News*, 1, 27–29. Cited on p. 45, 161.

Hothorn, T., Bretz, F., and Westfall, P. (2008), "Simultaneous inference in general parametric models," *Biometrical Journal*, 50, 346–363. Cited on p. 48, 49, 50, 69.

Hothorn, T., Bretz, F., Westfall, P., Heiberger, R. M., and Schützenmeister, A. (2010a), **multcomp**: Simultaneous Inference for General Linear Hypotheses, URL http://CRAN.R-project.org/package=multcomp, R package version 1.1-7. Cited on p. 53, 56, 66.

Hothorn, T., Hornik, K., van de Wiel, M., and Zeileis, A. (2010b), **coin**: Conditional Inference Procedures in a Permutation Test Framework, URL http://CRAN.R-project.org/package=coin, R package version 1.0-11. Cited on p. 127.

Hothorn, T., Hornik, K., van de Wiel, M. A., and Zeileis, A. (2006), "A Lego system for conditional inference," *The American Statistician*, 60, 257–263. Cited on p. 118, 137.

Hsu, J. C. (1996), *Multiple Comparisons*, London: Chapman & Hall. Cited on p. xiii, 11, 41, 85.

Hsu, J. C. and Berger, R. L. (1999), "Stepwise confidence intervals without multiplicity adjustment for dose-response and toxicity studies," *Journal of the American Statistical Association*, 94, 468–482. Cited on p. 30, 156.

Hsu, J. C. and Peruggia, M. (1994), "Graphical representations of Tukey's multiple comparison method," *Journal of Computational and Graphical Statistics*, 3, 143–161. Cited on p. 89.

Hsueh, H., Chen, J. J., and Kodell, R. L. (2003), "Comparison of methods for estimating the number of true null hypotheses in multiplicity testing," *Journal of Biopharmaceutical Statistics*, 13, 675–689. Cited on p. 35.

Hwang, I. K., Shih, W. J., and DeCani, J. S. (1990), "Group sequential designs using a family of Type I error probability spending functions," *Statistics in Medicine*, 9, 1439–1445. Cited on p. 144.

ICH (1998), ICH Topic E9: Notes for Guidance on Statistical Principles for Clinical Trials, International Conference on Harmonization, London, URL http://www.emea.europa.eu/pdfs/human/ich/036396en.pdf. Cited on p. 8.

Ihaka, R. and Gentleman, R. (1996), "R: A language for data analysis and graphics," *Journal of Computational and Graphical Statistics*, 5, 299–314. Cited on p. xiv.

Jennison, C. and Turnbull, B. W. (2000), *Group Sequential Methods with Applications to Clinical Trials*, Boca Raton: Chapman and Hall. Cited on p. 141.

Kieser, M., Bauer, P., and Lehmacher, W. (1999), "Inference on multiple endpoints in clinical trials with adaptive interim analyses," *Biometrical Journal*, 41, 261–277. Cited on p. 151, 152.

Kleinbaum, D. G., Kupper, L. L., Muller, K. E., and Nizam, A. (1998), *Applied Regression Analysis and Other Multivariable Methods*, North Scituate, MA: Duxbury Press. Cited on p. 111, 113.

Korn, E. L., Troendle, J. F., McShane, L. M., and Simon, R. (2004), "Controlling the number of false discoveries: Application to high-dimensional genomic data," *Journal of Statistical Planning and Inference*, 124, 379–398. Cited on p. 14.

Kotz, S., Balakrishnan, N., and Johnson, N. L. (2000), *Continuous Multivariate Distributions. Volume 1: Models and Applications*, New York: Wiley. Cited on p. 44.

Kotz, S. and Nadarajah, S. (2004), *Multivariate t Distributions and Their Applications*, Cambridge: Cambridge University Press. Cited on p. 44.

Krishna, R. (2006), *Dose Optimization in Drug Development*, New York: Informa Healthcare. Cited on p. 100.

Lan, K. K. G. and DeMets, D. L. (1983), "Discrete sequential boundaries for clinical trials," *Biometrika*, 70, 659–663. Cited on p. 142.

Laska, E. M. and Meisner, M. J. (1989), "Testing whether an identified treatment is best," *Biometrics*, 45, 1139–1151. Cited on p. 22.

Lehmacher, W. and Wassmer, G. (1999), "Adaptive sample size calculations in group sequential trials," *Biometrics*, 55, 1286–1290. Cited on p. 152.

Lehmann, E. L. (1957a), "A theory of some multiple decision problems I," *The Annals of Mathematical Statistics*, 28, 1–25. Cited on p. 11.

Lehmann, E. L. (1957b), "A theory of some multiple decision problems II," *The Annals of Mathematical Statistics*, 28, 547–572. Cited on p. 11.

Lehmann, E. L. (1986), *Testing Statistical Hypotheses*, New York: Wiley. Cited on p. 18.

Lehmann, E. L. and Romano, J. P. (2005), "Generalizations of the familywise error rate," *The Annals of Statistics*, 33, 1138–1154. Cited on p. 13.

Liu, W. (2010), *Simultaneous Inference for Regression*, Boca Raton: Taylor and Francis. Cited on p. 12, 114.

Liu, W., Jamshidian, M., and Zhang, Y. (2004), "Multiple comparison of several linear regression models," *Journal of the American Statistical Association*, 99, 395–403. Cited on p. 112.

Liu, W., Jamshidian, M., Zhang, Y., Bretz, F., and Han, X. (2007a), "Some new methods for the comparison of two linear regression models," *Journal of Statistical Planning and Inference*, 137, 57–67. Cited on p. 112, 113.

Liu, Y. and Hsu, J. (2009), "Testing for efficacy in primary and secondary endpoints by partitioning decision paths," *Journal of the American Statistical Association*, 104, 1661–1670. Cited on p. 30.

Liu, Y., Hsu, J. C., and Ruberg, S. (2007b), "Partition testing in dose-response studies with multiple endpoints," *Pharmaceutical Statistics*, 6, 181–192. Cited on p. 30.

Marcus, R. (1976), "The power of some tests of the equality of normal means against an ordered alternative," *Biometrika*, 63, 177–183. Cited on p. 103, 104, 105, 106, 157.

Marcus, R., Peritz, E., and Gabriel, K. R. (1976), "On closed testing procedures with special reference to ordered analysis of variance," *Biometrika*, 63, 655–660. Cited on p. 11, 23, 25, 78.

Maurer, W., Hothorn, L., and Lehmacher, W. (1995), "Multiple comparisons in drug clinical trials and preclinical assays: a-priori ordered hypotheses," in *Biometrie in der chemisch-pharmazeutischen Industrie*, ed. J. Vollmar, Stuttgart: Fischer Verlag, pp. 3–18. Cited on p. 28.

Maurer, W. and Mellein, B. (1988), "On new multiple test procedures based on independent p-values and the assessment of their power," in *Multiple Hypothesenprüfung - Multiple Hypotheses Testing*, eds. P. Bauer, G. Hommel, and E. Sonnemann, Heidelberg: Springer, pp. 48–66. Cited on p. 16.

Mehta, C. R., Bauer, P., Posch, M., and Brannath, W. (2007), "Repeated confidence intervals for adaptive group sequential trials," *Statistics in Medicine*, 26, 5422–5433. Cited on p. 149.

Müller, H. H. and Schäfer, H. (2001), "Adaptive group sequential designs for clinical trials: combining the advantages of adaptive and of classical group sequential approaches," *Biometrics*, 57, 886–891. Cited on p. 148, 151.

Naik, U. D. (1975), "Some selection rules for comparing p processes with a standard," *Communications in Statistics*, 4, 519–535. Cited on p. 78.

O'Brien, P. C. and Fleming, T. R. (1979), "A multiple testing procedure for clinical trials," *Biometrics*, 5, 549–556. Cited on p. 141, 142, 144.

Parsons, N. (2010), **asd**: Simulations for Adaptive Seamless Designs, URL http://CRAN.R-project.org/package=asd, R package version 1.0. Cited on p. 140, 153.

Parsons, N., Friede, T., Todd, S., Valdes-Marquez, E., Chataway, J., Nicholas, R., and Stallard, N. (2010), "An R package for implementing simulations for seamless phase II/III clinical trials using early outcomes for treatment selection," (submitted). Cited on p. 153.

Patel, H. I. (1991), "Comparison of treatments in a combination therapy trial," *Journal of Biopharmaceutical Statistics*, 1, 171–183. Cited on p. 23.

Petrondas, D. A. and Gabriel, K. R. (1983), "Multiple comparisons by rerandomization," *Journal of the American Statistical Association*, 78, 949–957. Cited on p. 133.

Piepho, H.-P. (2004), "An algorithm for a letter-based representation of all-pairwise comparisons," *Journal of Computational and Graphical Statistics*, 13, 456–466. Cited on p. 66, 87.

Pinheiro, J., Bornkamp, B., and Bretz, F. (2006a), "Design and analysis of dose finding studies combining multiple comparisons and modeling procedures," *Journal of Biopharmaceutical Statistics*, 16, 639–656. Cited on p. 157.

Pinheiro, J., Bretz, F., and Branson, M. (2006b), "Analysis of dose-response studies: Modeling approaches." in *Dose Finding in Drug Development.*, ed. N. Ting, New York: Springer Verlag, pp. 146–171. Cited on p. 159.

Pocock, S. J. (1977), "Group sequential methods in the design and analysis of clinical trials," *Biometrika*, 64, 191–199. Cited on p. 141, 142, 144.

Pollard, K. S., Gilbert, H. N., Ge, Y., Taylor, S., and Dudoit, S. (2010), **multtest**: Resampling-based Multiple Hypothesis Testing, URL http://CRAN.R-project.org/package=multtest, R package version 2.4.0. Cited on p. 137.

Posch, M., König, F., Branson, M., Brannath, W., Dunger-Baldauf, C., and Bauer, P. (2005), "Testing and estimation in flexible group sequential designs with adaptive treatment selection," *Statistics in Medicine*, 24, 3697–3714. Cited on p. 151.

Proschan, M., Lan, K. K. G., and Wittes, J. T. (2006), *Statistical Monitoring of Clinical Trials - A Unified Approach*, New York: Springer. Cited on p. 141.

Proschan, M. A. and Hunsberger, S. A. (1995), "Designed extension of studies based on conditional power," *Biometrics*, 51, 1315–1324. Cited on p. 151.

Ramsey, P. H. (1978), "Power differences between pairwise multiple comparisons," *Journal of the American Statistical Association*, 73, 479–487. Cited on p. 16.

Romano, J. P. and Wolf, M. (2005), "Exact and approximate stepdown methods for multiple hypothesis testing," *Journal of the American Statistical Association*, 100, 94–108. Cited on p. 28.

Rosenthal, R. and Rubin, D. B. (1983), "Ensemble-adjusted p-values," *Psychological Bulletin*, 94, 540–541. Cited on p. 35.

Rousseeuw, P., Croux, C., Todorov, V., Ruckstuhl, A., Salibian-Barrera, M., Verbeke, T., and Maechler, M. (2009), **robustbase**: Basic Robust Statistics, URL http://CRAN.R-project.org/package=robustbase, R package version 0.5-0-1. Cited on p. 110.

Rousseeuw, P. J. and Leroy, A. M. (2003), *Robust Regression and Outlier Detection*, New York: John Wiley & Sons. Cited on p. 52.

Roy, S. N. (1953), "On a heuristic method of test construction and its use in multivariate analysis," *Annals of Mathematical Statistics*, 24, 220–238. Cited on p. 20.

Roy, S. N. and Bose, R. C. (1953), "Simultaneous confidence interval estimation," *Annals of Mathematical Statistics*, 24, 513–536. Cited on p. 20.

Royen, T. (1991), "Generalized maximum range tests for pairwise comparisons of several populations," *Biometrical Journal*, 31, 905–929. Cited on p. 95.

Ruberg, S. J. (1995a), "Dose-response studies. I. Some design considerations," *Journal of Biopharmaceutical Statistics*, 5, 1–14. Cited on p. 100, 161.

Ruberg, S. J. (1995b), "Dose-response studies. II. Analysis and interpretation," *Journal of Biopharmaceutical Statistics*, 5, 15–42. Cited on p. 100.

Salib, E. and Hillier, V. (1997), "A case-control study of smoking and Alzheimer's disease," *International Journal of Geriatric Psychiatry*, 12, 295–300. Cited on p. 118, 123.

Samuel-Cahn, E. (1996), "Is the Simes' improved Bonferroni procedure conservative?" *Biometrika*, 83, 928–933. Cited on p. 37.

Sarkar, S. and Chang, C. K. (1997), "Simes' method for multiple hypothesis testing with positively dependent test statistics," *Journal of the American Statistical Association*, 92, 1601–1608. Cited on p. 38.

Sarkar, S. K. (1998), "Some probability inequalities for censored MTP_2 random variables: A proof of the Simes conjecture," *The Annals of Statistics*, 26, 494–504. Cited on p. 38.

Sarkar, S. K., Snapinn, S., and Wang, W. (1995), "On improving the min test for the analysis of combination drug trials," *Journal of Statistical Computation and Simulation*, 51, 197–213, correction: 60, (1998) 180–181. Cited on p. 23.

Schmidli, H., Bretz, F., Racine, A., and Maurer, W. (2006), "Confirmatory seamless phase II/III clinical trials with hypotheses selection at interim: Applications and practical considerations," *Biometrical Journal*, 48, 635–643. Cited on p. 152.

Schweder, T. and Spjøtvoll, E. (1982), "Plots of p-values to evaluate many tests simultaneously," *Biometrika*, 69, 493–502. Cited on p. 35.

Searle, S. R. (1971), *Linear Models*, New York: John Wiley & Sons. Cited on p. 41, 44.

Seeger, P. (1968), "A note on a method for the analysis of significance en masse," *Technometrics*, 10, 586–593. Cited on p. 13.

Senn, S. and Bretz, F. (2007), "Power and sample size when multiple endpoints are considered," *Pharmaceutical Statistics*, 6, 161–170. Cited on p. 16.

Serfling, R. J. (1980), *Approximation Theorems of Mathematical Statistics*, New York: John Wiley & Sons. Cited on p. 49, 50.

Shaffer, J. P. (1980), "Control of directional errors with stagewise multiple test procedures," *The Annals of Statistics*, 8, 1342–1347. Cited on p. 17.

Shaffer, J. P. (1986), "Modified sequentially rejective multiple test procedures," *Journal of the American Statistical Association*, 81, 826–831. Cited on p. 28, 34, 63, 95, 99, 100.

Šidák, Z. (1967), "Rectangular confidence regions for the means of multivariate normal distributions," *Journal of the American Statistical Association*, 62, 626–633. Cited on p. 34.

Simes, R. J. (1986), "An improved Bonferroni procedure for multiple tests of significance," *Biometrika*, 73, 751–754. Cited on p. 35, 37.

Solorzano, E. and Spurrier, J. D. (1999), "One-sided simultaneous comparisons with more than one control," *Journal of Statistical Computation and Simulation*, 63, 37–46. Cited on p. 77.

Sonnemann, E. (1982), "Allgemeine Lösungen multipler Testprobleme," *EDV in Medizin und Biologie*, 13, 120–128, translated by H. Finner and reprinted in: Sonnemann, E. (2008), "General solutions to multiple testing problems," *Biometrical Journal*, 50, 641–656. Cited on p. 11.

Sonnemann, E. and Finner, H. (1988), "Vollständigkeitssätze für multiple Testprobleme," in *Multiple Hypothesenprüfung - Multiple Hypotheses Testing*, eds. P. Bauer, G. Hommel, and E. Sonnemann, Heidelberg: Springer, pp. 121–135. Cited on p. 20.

Sorić, B. (1989), "Statistical "discoveries" and effect size estimation," *Journal of the American Statistical Association*, 84, 608–610. Cited on p. 13.

Spurrier, J. D. and Solorzano, E. (2004), "Multiple comparisons with more than one control," in *Recent Developments in Multiple Comparison Procedures*, eds. Y. Benjamini, F. Bretz, and S. Sarkar, volume 47 of *IMS Lecture Notes - Monograph Series*, pp. 119–128. Cited on p. 77.

Stefansson, G., Kim, W. C., and Hsu, J. C. (1988), "On confidence sets in multiple comparisons," in *Statistical Decision Theory and Related Topics IV*, eds. S. S. Gupta and J. O. Berger, New York: Academic Press, pp. 89–104. Cited on p. 11, 29.

Stewart, W. H. and Ruberg, S. (2000), "Detecting dose-response with contrasts," *Statistics in Medicine*, 19, 913–921. Cited on p. 157.

Storey, J. D. (2002), "A direct approach to false discovery rates," *Jornal of the Royal Statistical, Society B*, 64, 479–498. Cited on p. 35.

Storey, J. D. (2003), "The positive false discovery rate: A Bayesian interpretation and the q-value," *The Annals of Statistics*, 31, 2013–2035. Cited on p. 13.

Strassburger, K. and Bretz, F. (2008), "Compatible simultaneous lower confidence bounds for the Holm procedure and other Bonferroni based closed tests," *Statistics in Medicine*, 27, 4914–4927. Cited on p. 19, 28, 31, 34, 81.

Strassburger, K., Bretz, F., and Finner, H. (2007), "Ordered multiple comparisons with the best and their applications to dose-response studies," *Biometrics*, 63, 1143–1151. Cited on p. 30, 157.

Strassburger, K., Bretz, F., and Hochberg, Y. (2004), "Compatible confidence intervals for intersection union tests involving two hypotheses," in *Recent Developments in Multiple Comparison Procedures*, eds. Y. Benjamini, F. Bretz, and S. Sarkar, Beachwood, Ohio: Institute of Mathematical Statistics, volume 47 of *IMS Lecture Notes - Monograph Series*, pp. 129–142. Cited on p. 19, 23, 30.

Strasser, H. and Weber, C. (1999), "On the asymptotic theory of permutation statistics," *Mathematical Methods of Statistics*, 8, 220–250. Cited on p. 137.

Takeuchi, K. (1973), *Studies in Some Aspects of Theoretical Foundations of Statistical Data Analysis*, Tokyo: Toyo Keizai Shinposha, (in Japanese). Cited on p. 29.

Takeuchi, K. (2010), "Basic ideas and concepts for multiple comparison procedures," *Biometrical Journal*, (in press). Cited on p. 29.

Tamhane, A. C., Dunnett, C. W., Green, J. W., and Wetherington, J. D. (2001), "Multiple test procedures for identifying the maximum safe dose," *Journal of the American Statistical Association*, 96, 835–843. Cited on p. 156.

Tamhane, A. C., Hochberg, Y., and Dunnett, C. W. (1996), "Multiple test procedures for dose finding," *Biometrics*, 52, 21–37. Cited on p. 156.

Tamhane, A. C. and Logan, B. (2006), "Multiple comparison procedures for dose response studies," in *Dose Finding in Drug Development.*, ed. N. Ting, New York: Springer Verlag, pp. 172–183. Cited on p. 157.

Ting, N. (2006), *Dose Finding in Drug Development*, New York: Springer. Cited on p. 100.

Tong, Y. L. (1980), *Probability Inequalities in Multivariate Distributions*, New York: Academic Press. Cited on p. 34.

Tong, Y. L. (1990), *The Multivariate Normal Distribution*, New York: Springer Verlag. Cited on p. 44.

Troendle, J. (1995), "A stepwsie resampling method of multiple hypothesis testing," *Journal of the American Statistical Association*, 90, 370–378. Cited on p. 127.

Troendle, J., Korn, E., and McShane, L. (2004), "An example of slow convergence of the bootstrap in high dimensions," *The American Statistician*, 58, 25–29. Cited on p. 140.

Tukey, J. W. (1953), The Problem of Multiple Comparisons, unpublished manuscript reprinted in: The Collected Works of John W. Tukey, Volume 8, 1994, H. I. Braun (Ed.), Chapman and Hall, New York. Cited on p. 83, 100.

Tukey, J. W. (1977), *Exploratory Data Analysis*, Reading, Mass: Addison-Wesley. Cited on p. 53.

Tukey, J. W., Ciminera, J. L., and Heyse, J. F. (1985), "Testing the statistical certainty of a response to increasing doses of a drug," *Biometrics*, 41, 295–301. Cited on p. 157.

van der Laan, M. J., Dudoit, S., and Pollard, K. S. (2004), "Augmentation procedures for control of the generalized family-wise error rate and tail probabilities for the proportion of false positives," *Statistical Applications in Genetics and Molecular Biology*, 3(1). Cited on p. 14.

Vandemeulebroecke, M. (2009), **adaptTest**: Adaptive Two-stage Tests, URL http://CRAN.R-project.org/package=adaptTest, R package version 1.0. Cited on p. 153.

Venables, W. N. and Ripley, B. D. (2002), *Modern Applied Statistics with S*, New York: Springer. Cited on p. 82, 83.

Victor, N. (1982), "Exploratory data-analysis and clinical research," *Methods of Information in Medicine*, 21, 53–54. Cited on p. 13.

Wang, S. J., O'Neill, R. T., and Hung, H. M. J. (2007), "Approaches to evaluation of treatment effect in randomized clinical trials with genomic subset," *Pharmaceutical Statistics*, 6, 227–244. Cited on p. 152.

Wang, S. K. and Tsiatis, A. A. (1987), "Approximately optimal one parameter boundaries for group sequential trials," *Biometrics*, 43, 193–199. Cited on p. 142, 143, 144.

Wassmer, G. (1999), *Statistische Testverfahren für gruppensequentielle und adaptive Pläne in klinischen Studien. Theoretische Konzepte und deren praktische Umsetzung mit SAS*, Köln: Verlag Alexander Mönch. Cited on p. 141.

Wassmer, G. (2009), "Group sequential designs," in *Encyclopedia of Clinical Trials*, eds. R. D'Agostino, L. Sullivan, and J. Massaro, Hoboken: Wiley. Cited on p. 141.

Westfall, P. (2005), "Combining p-values," in *Encyclopedia of Biostatistics*, eds. P. Armitage and T. Colton, Chichester: Wiley, pp. 987–991. Cited on p. 22.

Westfall, P., Krishen, A., and Young, S. S. (1998), "Using prior information to allocate significance levels for multiple endpoints," *Statistics in Medicine*, 17, 2107–2119. Cited on p. 139.

Westfall, P., Tobias, R., and Bretz, F. (2000), Estimating directional error rates of stepwise multiple comparison methods using distributed computing and variance reduction, URL http://support.sas.com/rnd/app/papers/directional.pdf, Technical Report. Cited on p. 17.

Westfall, P. H. (1997), "Multiple testing of general contrasts using logical constraints and correlations," *Journal of the American Statistical Association*, 92, 299–306. Cited on p. 51, 63, 95, 98, 99, 100, 103, 104, 157.

Westfall, P. H. and Bretz, F. (2010), "Multiplicity in clinical trials," in *Encyclopedia of Biopharmaceutical Statistics*, ed. S. C. Chow, New York: Marcel Dekker Inc., (in press). Cited on p. 6, 15.

Westfall, P. H. and Krishen, A. (2001), "Optimally weighted, fixed sequence, and gatekeeping multiple testing procedures," *Journal of Statistical Planning and Inference*, 99, 25–40. Cited on p. 28.

Westfall, P. H., Kropf, S., and Finos, L. (2004), "Weighted FWE-controlling methods in high-dimensional situations," in *Recent Developments in Multiple Comparison Procedures*, eds. Y. Benjamini, F. Bretz, and S. Sarkar, Beachwood, Ohio: Institute of Mathematical Statistics, volume 47 of *IMS Lecture Notes - Monograph Series*, pp. 143–154. Cited on p. 35.

Westfall, P. H. and Tobias, R. D. (2007), "Multiple testing of general contrasts: Truncated closure and the extended Shaffer-Royen method," *Journal of the American Statistical Association*, 102, 487–494. Cited on p. 28, 34, 51, 63, 95.

Westfall, P. H., Tobias, R. D., Rom, D., Wolfinger, R. D., and Hochberg, Y. (1999), *Multiple Comparisons and Multiple Tests Using the SAS System*, Cary, NC: SAS Institute Inc. Cited on p. xiii, xvi, 16, 71, 113, 136.

Westfall, P. H. and Troendle, J. (2008), "Multiple testing with minimal assumptions," *Biometrical Journal*, 50, 745–755. Cited on p. 127, 130, 133.

Westfall, P. H. and Young, S. S. (1993), *Resampling-Based Multiple Testing*, New York: Wiley. Cited on p. xiii, 18, 19, 28, 100, 101, 127, 133.

Wiens, B. L. (2003), "A fixed sequence Bonferroni procedure for testing multiple endpoints," *Pharmaceutical Statistics*, 2, 211–215. Cited on p. 28.

Wiens, B. L. and Dmitrienko, A. (2005), "The fallback procedure for evaluating a single family of hypotheses," *Journal of Biopharmaceutical Statistics*, 15, 929–942. Cited on p. 28.

Williams, D. A. (1971), "A test for difference between treatment means when several dose levels are compared with a zero dose control," *Biometrics*, 27, 103–117. Cited on p. 103, 104, 105, 106, 157.

Wright, S. P. (1992), "Adjusted p-values for simultaneous inference," *Biometrics*, 48, 1005–1013. Cited on p. 18.

Yohai, V. J. (1987), "High breakdown-point and high efficiency estimates for regression," *The Annals of Statistics*, 15, 642–665. Cited on p. 110.

Zeileis, A. (2006), "Object-oriented computation of sandwich estimators," *Journal of Statistical Software*, 16, 1–16. Cited on p. 117.

Index

Underlined page numbers for the subject items below refer to those places in the book where the associated topic is introduced and/or discussed in detail.

Adaptive design, <u>150</u>
  p-value combination function, 151
  adaptTest, 153
  asd, 153
  Fisher's product test, 151
  Inverse normal combination test, 152
  Operational definition, 151
  Schematic diagram, 153
Adjusted p-value, 18
  multcomp, 60
Adverse event analysis, *see* Multiple
  comparison problems
All pairwise comparisons, *see* Multiple
  comparison problems, Tukey test
Analysis of covariance, 41, 101
Analysis of variance, 41, 52
  χ^2 test, 50, 60
  F test, 50, 60, 83, 109, 111
  Linear regression model, *see*
    Regression
  Mixed-effects model, 48, 52, 126
  One-way layout, 53, 71, 115
  Robust, 52, 110, 117
  Two-way layout, 82
Average power, *see* Power

Bonferroni inequality, 31
Bonferroni test, 4, 17, 23, <u>31</u>, 128
  Adjusted p-value, 5, 31
  Comparison to Simes test, 36
  multcomp, 61
  p.adjust function, 31
  Rejection region, 36
  Simultaneous confidence intervals,
    34, 65
  Weighted, 35
Bootstrap testing, 140

Closed test procedure, 26, *see also*
  Step-down test, Step-up test
  Closed Dunnett test, *see* Step-down
    test
  Closed Tukey test, <u>93</u>
    Comparison to other methods, 99
    multcomp, 98
    Schematic diagram, 96
    Truncated, 34, 95
Closure principle, <u>23</u>, 78, 93, 127, 129,
  134
  Adjusted p-value, 26
  Control of familywise error rate, 27
  Operational definition, 26
  Shortcut, 28, 79, 133
  Simultaneous confidence intervals, 28
  Visualization
    Parameter space, 23
    Schematic diagram, <u>24</u>, 25, 27, 33,
      81, 96, 130, 153
    Venn diagram, 24
Coherence, <u>20</u>, 21, 24, 26
Combined error rate, 16
Comparisons with a control, *see*
  Multiple comparison problems,
  Dunnett test
Conjunctive power, *see* Power
Consonance, <u>20</u>, 21
Contrasts, 42
  General, 103
  Modified Williams, *see* Trend test
  multcomp, 104
  Orthogonal, 93
  Other comparisons than contrasts,
    43, 121, 126
  Pairwise, 56, 75, 77, 101
  Treatment contrasts in R, 57, 116,
    122

Williams, *see* Trend test

Dataset, xvi
  alpha, 115
  alzheimer, 118
  biom, 162
  bodyfat, 108
  clinical, 124
  immer, 82
  litter, 101
  recovery, 71
  sbp, 113
  thuesen, 3, 42
  trees513, 125
  warpbreaks, 53
Directional error, 6, 12, <u>16</u>
Discrete data, *see* Sparse data
Disjunctive power, *see* Power
Dose response analysis, 99, 156, *see also*
  Trend test
  MCP-Mod procedure, 156
Dunnett test, <u>71</u>, 101
  Comparison to other methods, 81
  Contrast matrix, 75
  Correlation, 73
  Distribution, 72
  multcomp, 73
  Null hypothesis, 72
  Simultaneous confidence intervals, 74
  Step-down, *see* Step-down test
  Step-up, *see* Step-up test
  Test statistic, 72
  With covariates, 101

Effective number of tests, 128
Elementary null hypothesis, 11
Error rate, 11

Fallback procedure, 28
False discovery rate, 13
False negative, *see* Type II error
False positive, *see* Type I error
Family of hypotheses, 13, 15
Familywise error rate, <u>13</u>, 129
Fixed sequence test, 28
Free combinations, <u>19</u>
Function

aov, xvi, 53, 55, 60, 73, 82, 101, 106,
  115
asd.sim, 153
cld, 66, 88
contrMat, 55, 104–106
glht, 5, 46, 53–60, 73–75, 77, 84–86,
  90, 91, 106, 107, 109, 113, 116,
  117, 119
glht.mmc, 90, 91, 93
glm, 55, 118
gsCP, 148
gsDesign, 145, 146
gsProbability, 147
independence_test, 138, 139
lm, xvi, 45, 55, 108, 113
lmer, 126
lmrob, 110
mcp, 55, 73, 77, 84
MCPMod, 163
model.tables, 83
nlme, xvi
p.adjust, 31, 32, 39, 61, 63
pmvt, 45
sandwich, 117
survreg, 124
TukeyHSD, 85
uniroot, 46

Gatekeeping procedure, 28
General parametric model, <u>48</u>
  Adjusted *p*-value, 51
  Simultaneous confidence intervals, 51
Generalized familywise error rate, 13
Generalized linear model, 48, 52
Global null hypothesis, 14, 21
Group sequential design, <u>141</u>
  AGSDest, 149
  Average sample size, 142
  Error spending function, 142
  gsDesign, 145
  O'Brien-Fleming boundaries, 142,
    145
  Pocock boundaries, 142
  Wang-Tsiatis boundaries, 142

Hochberg procedure, 38
  Adjusted *p*-value, 38
  multcomp, 61

p.adjust function, 39
Holm procedure, 17, 19, 20, 32
    Adjusted p-value, 32
    Comparison to Hochberg procedure,
        38
    multcomp, 61
    p.adjust function, 32
    Weighted, 35
Hommel procedure, 38
    Comparison to Hochberg procedure,
        39
    multcomp, 61
    p.adjust function, 39

Individual power, see Power
Intersection union test, 22

Letter display, see Tukey test
Linear model, 42
    Simultaneous confidence intervals, 44
Logical constraints, see Restricted
    combinations

Many-to-one comparisons, see Multiple
    comparison problems, Dunnett test
Marginal p-value, 4, 18
    multcomp, 61
max-t test, 21, 78, 130, 133, see also
    Union intersection test
Mean-mean comparison plot, 89
min test, 22, see also Intersection union
    test
min-p test, 130
multcomp package, see also Package
    cld, 66
    coef, 55
    confint, 64
    contrMat, 55, 104
    glht, 5, 46, 53
    mcp, 55
    modelparm, 55
    plot, 64
    print, 57
    summary, 59
    vcov, 55
Multiple comparison problems
    Adaptive design, 150, see also
        Adaptive design

Adverse event analysis, 128, 131, 137
All pairwise comparisons, 53, 82, 116,
    124, see also Tukey test
    Comparisons with a control, 70, see
        also Dunnett test
    Comparisons with several controls, 77
    Dose response, see Dose response
        analysis
    General contrasts, 103
    Group sequential design, 141, see also
        Group sequential design
    Many-to-one comparisons, 72, see
        also Dunnett test
    Multiple endpoint analysis, 128, 139
    Repeated hypothesis testing, 140
    Safety analysis, 128, 131, 137
    Simultaneous confidence bands, 111
    Subgroup analysis, 118
    Variable selection, 108
Multiple comparison procedure, 15
    Construction methods, 20
Multiple endpoint analysis, see Multiple
    comparison problems
Multiple testing, 7
Multiplicity problem, 1–3, 6
Multivariate t distribution, 43, 59, 72
Multivariate normal distribution, 59
    asymptotic, 43, 50

One-sided studentized range test, see
    Tukey test

p.adjust function, 31, 61
Package, xvi
    adaptTest, 153, 181
    AGSDest, 149, 172
    asd, 140, 153, 155, 176
    coin, 127, 137–139, 174
    datasets, 53
    DoseFinding, 157, 160, 162, 168
    gsDesign, 140, 141, 145, 148, 149,
        167
    HH, 65, 86, 90, 93, 173
    ISwR, xvi, 3, 170
    lme4, 126, 167
    MASS, xvi, 82
    multcomp, xiv, xvi, xvii, 4–6, 28,
        31, 34, 41, 45–48, 51, 53, 54, 59,

62–64, 66, 69–71, 73–75, 77, 78, 80,
    81, 84, 85, 87, 93, 95, 98, 101, 103,
    104, 106, 109, 113, 114, 116, 123,
    174
multtest, 137, 177
mvtnorm, 45, 63, 65, 161, 172
robustbase, 110, 177
sandwich, 117
stats, 31, 61, 85
survival, 124
Partitioning principle, 18, <u>29</u>
    Visualization, 30
Per-comparison error rate, 12
Permutation test, 127
    coin, 137
    Fisher's exact test, 128, 131
    Joint exchangeability assumption,
        130
    Multiple-sample problem, 127
    Subset pivotality, 133, 134, 136
    Two-sample problem, 129
Positive false discovery rate, 13
Power, <u>15</u>
    Average, 15
    Conjunctive, 16
    Disjunctive, 16, 155
    Individual, 15
Proportion of false positives, 14

Regression, <u>42</u>, 52
    Logistic, 118, 126
    Multiple linear, 108
    Non-linear, 159
    Simple linear, 3, 42, 45, 111
Repeated hypothesis testing, *see*
    Multiple comparison problems
Reproducibility, 6
Resampling-based test, *see* Permutation
    test, Bootstrap test
Restricted combinations, <u>19</u>, 95, 135

Safety analysis, *see* Multiple
    comparison problems
Selection effect, 6
Shaffer procedure, 19, 34, 95, 99
    Comparison to other methods, 99
Shortcut procedure, *see* Closure
    principle

Sidák approach, 34, 122
Simes test, <u>35</u>
    Distributional assumptions, 37
    Rejection region, 36
Simultaneous confidence bands, 111
    Approximation, 113
Simultaneous confidence intervals, <u>18</u>,
    44, 81, 91, 121, 126
    multcomp, 64
Single-step test, <u>17</u>
Sparse data, 128, 130, 136
Step-down test, <u>17</u>
    Algorithm under free combinations,
        79
    Holm, *see* Holm procedure
    Shaffer, *see* Shaffer procedure
    Step-down Dunnett test, <u>77</u>, 80, 103
        Comparison to other methods, 81
        multcomp, 80
        Schematic diagram, 81
Step-up test, 17
    Hochberg, *see* Hochberg procedure
    Step-up Dunnett test, 78
Stepwise test procedure, <u>17</u>, 93
Strong control of error rates, 14
Studentized range test, *see* Tukey test
Subgroup analysis, *see* Multiple
    comparison problems
Subset pivotality, *see* Permutation test
Survival analysis, 48, 52, 124

Treatment contrasts, *see* Contrasts
Trend test, 103
    Contrast test, 103
        multcomp, 106
    MCP-Mod procedure, 156
    Modified Williams contrast test, 106
    One-sided studentized range test, *see*
        Tukey test
    Williams contrast test, 104
Truncated closed test, *see* Closed test
    procedure
Tukey test, <u>82</u>, 116, 124
    Closed Tukey test, *see* Closed test
        procedure
    Comparison to other methods, 99
    Contrast matrix, 56, 116
    Distribution, 84
    Generalized Tukey test, 93

Hypotheses, 53, 83
Letter display, 66, 87
multcomp, 55, 84
One-sided studentized range test, 85
Simultaneous confidence intervals, 64, 86, 118
Test statistics, 59, 83
`TukeyHSD` function, 85
Under heteroscedasticity, 114
`TukeyHSD` function, *see* Tukey test
Type I error, 7, <u>12</u>, *see also* Error Rate Inflation, 1
Type II error, <u>12</u>, 15, *see also* Power
Type III error, *see* Directional error

Unadjusted p-value, *see* Marginal p-value
Union intersection test, <u>20</u>, 24

Variable selection, *see* Multiple comparison problems

Weak control of error rates, 14

Printed in the United States
by Baker & Taylor Publisher Services